Praise for Boomer Be Well

Susan has written the definitive, "must-have" guide for Boomers to live with health and vitality. Buy this book for yourself and someone you care about; you'll both be glad you did.

—Carol Fenster
100 Best Gluten-Free Recipes

Boomer Be Well! is a delightful book and sure to be helpful to Baby Boomers interested in maximizing the quality of their life. Susan Piergeorge writes with an easy style that will draw in even the most health-phobic Boomer and have them taking a second look at what's possible and the huge benefits of taking responsibility for their health. Plus, she takes you step by step from where you are to where you could be. Enjoy!

—Ruth DeBusk, PhD, RD
It's Not Just Your Genes!

Piergeorge has just written a Boomer Manifesto. What a great go-to, resourcy-sort-of-guide—it contains vital nutrition and lifestyle info that boomers need for tackling life's inevitabilities.

—David W. Grotto, RD, LDN
101 Optimal Life Foods and *101 Foods That Could Save Your Life!*

I0862639

BOOMER BE WELL!

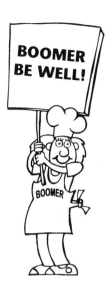

BOOMER BE WELL!

*Rebel Against Aging through
Food, Nutrition and Lifestyle*

Susan M. Piergeorge, MS, RD

The information in this book is intended to provide suggestions and
insight into health maintenance. It is not intended to replace the services
of a qualified healthcare practitioner. It is essential for the reader to seek
medical attention if they are experiencing a health issue or concern.
Any adverse effect or reaction from information in this book is the sole
responsibility of the reader and not that of the author or publisher.

Editor: John Maling, Editing by John
Interior Book Design: Ronnie Moore, WESType Publishing Services, Inc.
Cover Design and Charts: Nick Zellinger, NZ Graphics
Illustrations: Don Sidle
Book Shepherds: Judith Briles and Katherine Carol

ISBN 978-0-9846006-0-1
Library of Congress Control Number: 2010915992

1. Nutrition   2. Health   3. Food   4. Lifestyle
5. Aging   6. Recipes

Published in USA by

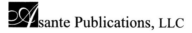sante Publications, LLC

Printed in the United States

This book is dedicated to my deceased parents,
Andrew and Helen.
I would not be who I am
without their faith, love and integrity.

Acknowledgments

I owe a great deal to my brother, Jeffry, who inspired me to write in the first place.

To my many friends, family, and colleagues I say thank you for continued support, guidance, and interest.

To Ruth DeBusk, PhD, RD, Shelly Case, RD, Roberta Larson Duyff, MS, RD, FADA, CFCS, Carol Fenster, David Grotto, RD, LDN, Steve Eunpu, Marjorie Geiser, MBA, RD, NSCA-CPT, Erica Gradwell, MS, RD, Marla Heller, MS, RD, Jan Patenaude, RD, CLT, Anthony Sepe, C. Alan Titchenal, PhD, CNS, and Tom Wnorowski, PhD, I thank you all for your expertise and insight.

To my editor John Maling, along with Book Shepherd's Judith Briles and Katherine Carol, for making it happen.

To Ronnie Lynn Moore of WESType Publishing Services, Inc. for putting it all together.

To my cover and interior designers Don Sidle and Nick Zellinger for their innovation and creativity. To Michael Shuck of Adapt Merch, Inc. for his artistic talent.

To Dr. Michael Taravella, I am eternally grateful to you for restoring my vision to be able to literally see this come to fruition.

To FedEx Office for fixing things in mere minutes.

Table of Contents

Introduction

Ah, the Baby Boomer generation. Born between 1946 and 1964, we are 75+ million strong. We have much to be grateful for, as we have grown up, worked hard, and want to enjoy the rewards of those efforts. Living life to the fullest is what our generation is all about. **Staying active and aging gracefully is part of the plan.** We are *not* going to let age slow us down.

There is plenty of evidence to show that if we take care of ourselves now, chances are we will have a better quality of life in the future. We can start at any time to reap the benefits of well health.

Many of us don't really think much about what we put into our bodies let alone what we do with and to them. All too often it takes a wake-up call to start thinking about our health. Developing and maintaining a healthy lifestyle starts with the desire and willingness to commit to making changes. It is about investing in and thinking of you and your well being. It is not about deprivation and difficult-to-follow regimens.

Often people strive to make lifestyle changes with good intentions and things end up not going the way they planned. There are a few reasons for that. One is called life, with its twists and unexpected turns. The other is that we are all different and need to appreciate that. Going on a one size fits all regimen may work temporarily. However, after we have reached "the goal," has anything really been learned to incorporate true lifestyle solutions for your life? Far too often we go for the fastest fix and put the long term planning aside. And the cycle goes on and on. We boomers have been around and seen a lot of fads come and go.

If you want to make changes to improve your health, incorporate realistic goals. Any type of change is more effective if it has variety, includes some fun, and does not necessarily cost a lot of money. Use the tools you already have. They are right there inside you. Get them out of storage. Remember—the journey is part of the destination.

Our lifestyles have certainly changed from when we were children. Our global culture has become much more connected, with even our health statistics aligning. Maintaining health is becoming a matter of fiscal responsibility. Many in the health and economic sectors are keeping a close watch on just how connected our health statistics are in relation to global economics.

Body type and genetic makeup is unique to each individual. The study of DNA and what science is revealing about genetics is becoming more prevalent. The science of nutritional genomics is evolving and will likely grow to play a larger part in modalities of individualized healthcare regimens. This science is something we will likely take a greater interest in as time progresses. Nanotechnology is a new science that will likely affect us in many aspects of our lives, including food, nutrition and healthcare.

Influences such as advertising and marketing have played and continue to play a huge role in everyday decisions, from how we eat to how we live. Becoming your own safety advocate is important when it comes to purchasing products related to your health.

Credible sources for health information can be difficult to find. A discussion of different types of practitioners in nutrition and exercise, along with their education and credentialing requirements is presented.

As individuals become more aware of strategies to improve their health, many have turned to using supplements. This industry continues to grow at a huge pace. The 1994 Dietary Supplement

Health and Education Act (DSHEA) enabled the US Food and Drug Administration (FDA) to provide guidelines to protect the public from any false or misleading claims made by supplement manufacturers. This became an initial step for the FDA in developing guidelines.

The safety of our foods along with how we handle and prepare them is an important component in our health. We will review suggestions on how to shop, prepare and store foods in our home. Shopping on a budget and how to understand a food label will be explored.

Provided in this book are easy instructions for calculating daily caloric needs along with protein, carbohydrate and fat recommendations. Also presented are the basics of protein, carbohydrates, fats and fiber, what they are, and how to understand why each group is a necessary part of daily eating.

Understanding how to estimate the content of foods and portion sizes can be a simple task. It can assist us all when we are dining out or buying prepared foods. Tips for learning how to estimate what is in our foods along with estimating portion sizes are reviewed.

The benefits of exercise and strategies to incorporate it into our daily lives are given. A simple calculation for energy expenditure is also provided.

Powerful compounds known as antioxidants and their potential in maintaining well health are explored. Of course, no book with any reference to food is without a few recipes included. Recipes in each section incorporate compounds and foods that may alleviate symptoms and reduce risk factors for each specific condition.

The aging process tends to make us all become a little more aware of symptoms we were once able to more easily ignore. Studies have shown that a few simple lifestyle adjustments may help alleviate conditions and accompanying symptoms that occur as we age, such as arthritis, cardiovascular disease, diabetes, eye health and osteoporosis. Something as simple as a restful night of sleep may play a role in risk reduction in some of these conditions.

Developing a REAL—**R**ealistic **E**ating **A**nd **L**ifestyle—approach is about enjoying life happily, healthfully while not doing without. Shifting our mindset is the key. Start thinking OF yourself FOR yourself. **And don't forget the word "life" in lifestyle!**

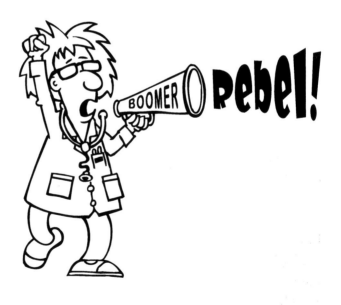

Chapter 1

Our Generation

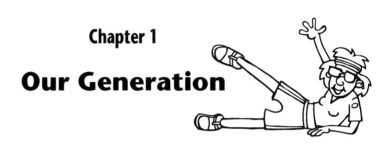

The Age We Live In

We live in some pretty incredible times. Think about all the magnificent events and changes we boomers have experienced. Men landing on the moon, miracles in medicine and technological changes we once thought of as science fiction are now a reality. With that, our lifestyles have transformed as well and are a result of this progress. We've adapted to cell phones, computers, televisions, social networking. We've also adopted new eating habits. A double meat patty burger with cheese, bacon, a side order of large fries and a 32-ounce beverage is a common menu item at many fast food restaurants. That meal in itself can be well beyond an individual's daily caloric needs.

Our lifestyles are much more sedentary than when we were children. The television set was fairly new, and that was only the beginning. Technology now takes care of things for us. We weren't born with a cell phone in our hands. Convenience was gradually incorporated into our lives.

We also have information available 24 hours a day. In fact, we have so much information coming at us it can be dizzying to process it all. One day we read or hear something about an incredible breakthrough in nutrition or wellness, then a year or two later, it has been found to be not so incredible after all. Many of us are looking for simple solutions to take better care of ourselves. An endless number of products out there claim to do just that—courtesy of your cash and/or credit card. What hooks us in is the packaging of all these products.

Many times, however, those products end up not performing up to the promised expectations. Plenty of people have purchased fitness equipment that ends up either becoming a new clothes hanger or dust collector. Many also spend a lot of money on miracle supplements that they can get right in the foods they eat (depending on what they choose to eat). We have become accustomed to *if a little of something is good, a larger dose must be better*. This is not necessarily true when it comes to our health. One would think all of this progress and convenience would make us all healthier and more likely to have an easier life. However, for many of us this progress seems to have taken away more of our time and added more stress into our lives.

We can fester about what's right or wrong with all of this or we can make things work to our advantage. Getting back to the basics is really the simpler way to go: behavior modification, good nutrition, reasonable caloric intake, exercise, and stress management. Develop your own set of P's—make yourself the *priority*, become *passionate* about your health and well being, create a *pattern*, be *persistent*, and practice *patience*.

A Global Effect

Society's move toward more convenience and technology and less physical activity has come at a very "hefty" price. Statistically, we are all gaining weight, and it's not just in the United States anymore. Globally ~ (approximately) 1.1 billion adults are considered overweight or obese, and 10 percent of children are as well.[1] Even nations such as Japan and China are experiencing an increase in obesity. In China, for example, one in every five people is overweight or obese.[2] Accompanying this "globesity" are increased risk factors of cardiovascular disease, cancer, diabetes, respiratory problems, and sleep disturbances.[3] Our generation has also developed a condition known as *metabolic syndrome.*

The majority of these ailments are linked to lifestyle. How has the status of our health come to this with all the numerous tools, diets, and everything else available to make life easier? Perhaps that is part of the confusion, thus part of the problem. We have way too many choices for everything. Often we select the easiest and least laborious option. It really should come as no surprise that if we eat more and expend less physical energy, we are going to weigh more. We may not feel the effects of that extra weight initially, but over time, it will manifest itself in our bodies. Thus, accompanying illnesses can occur.

Obesity and its related complications also create an economic impact. A reduction in worker productivity and quality of life can stem from this condition. Adding to the reduction in worker productivity are increases in the costs of healthcare. The health-care costs of obesity and its related conditions are greater than those related to smoking or drinking. In a 2006 EU-US Conference on Diet, Physical Activity and Health, statistics revealed that obesity accounts for up to seven percent of direct healthcare costs and if the current trend continues, costs will further increase.[4] Most importantly, obesity has been shown to potentially reduce lifespan. This trend does not have to continue.

We live in an age where information abounds in regards to health and wellness. It is not necessary for us to wait until our healthcare practitioner tells us our health is in jeopardy. Many health conditions can be treated and reduced in severity with a few simple lifestyle changes. A lot of individuals live in what I call "denial of diagnosis." Many conditions such as diabetes and cardio-vascular disease can be treated when diagnosed. Many people are prescribed medication. Along with the medication, a prescription of proper nutrition, regular exercise, and stress management is usually given. Usually—and unfortunately not in all cases—some type of education should be provided to assist an individual in treating their condition. More often than not, many do not consistently manage their condition or health. For whatever reason, they do not want to acknowledge they need to make some changes. An individual might take their medication and that is all.

Medication, however, is only one component of improving health. And with medication, side effects may occur and body chemistry may be changed. These changes can also have an impact on mental, physical and nutritional status. Let's also remember they are not cheap. Many clients I have worked with who were diagnosed with, for example, diabetes or cardiovascular disease at a younger age chose to ignore it. They took their medication, but made no other lifestyle changes, such as diet, exercise, smoking cessation, etc. Decades later, they felt the toll of their denial. Some experienced loss of eyesight or a limb with diabetes; a heart attack or stroke with cardiovascular disease. Their bodies could only handle so much for so long. I truly believe every situation has a solution. The first thing we can and need to do is to become conscious about ourselves. That in itself is a huge step for many. This should be THE priority for us.

An Era in Eating

In the 1990s and early 2000s a new era in eating emerged—large portions and a "supersize me" mentality. It skewed the way we view portion sizes, and it also created a trend to larger waistlines to say the least.

Because we have adapted to larger servings, the majority of people don't have a clue as to what a recommended serving is or looks like, let alone their daily caloric needs. Eating involves sensory and physical satisfaction. Social interaction is also an activity we have paired with it. Eating also has a purpose—nutrition.

Food turns into compounds in our bodies which provide nourishment. For some reason, we have veered from the basic understanding of this to having become visually oriented in regards to what we eat. We eat with our eyes, and choose what looks more delicious. It is not easy to resist the visual temptation of some foods, especially when they are put into a "package" or "bargain" meal.

Accompanying those large food portions are beverages. Many of them are supersized as well. We may not even think of beverages having calories, but many do. In the United States, 20+ percent of caloric intake is from beverages.[5] Black coffee and tea have become a rarity, as new items such as Frappuccinos, Grande Mochas and Chai Teas have come along and can contain up to 500 calories per serving.

There is also a multitude of energy drinks popping up on a regular basis. While many of these new and improved beverages are touted as "nutritional energy," it is important to read the labels and servings per container. While some are fortified with vitamins, minerals, and other potentially healthy ingredients, they may also include sugar, caffeine and, in some cases fat.

Water without any added ingredients has no calories and is something our bodies need on a daily basis. A simple switch to drinking more plain water with or between meals will not only hydrate our bodies, it may reduce our appetite and can also reduce caloric intake. That step in itself can be an easy solution if weight loss or maintenance is a goal.

Today, more foods are processed and stripped of their nutritional content. Part of this is due to mass production, "conveyor belt" farming practices and environmental pollution. Foods that withstand processing, production and transportation, along with having a shelf life of weeks to months is quite amazing. Food additives and preservatives are also part of our "progress." Adding preservatives to keep foods fresh, emulsifiers to maintain product consistency, and other ingredients added for various reasons has led to a number of people developing either a sensitivity or reaction to these products.

Some of us may not realize we have a reaction to foods; the response can be as subtle as a mild headache or a tickle in the back of the throat. Other reactions are more severe such as difficulty breathing, breaking out in a rash, or difficulty digesting the food product. If you experience these types of symptoms on a regular basis with certain foods and/or supplements discuss this with your healthcare practitioner. For some, reactions can be fatal. Nowadays there are a lot of tests that can be performed and solutions that can be provided.

To assist the consumer, many food manufacturers are now stating on their labels that their products contain certain additives or ingredients that have been shown to cause allergic reactions. A number of manufacturers do add some of the nutrition lost in processing back to the food product. Some are also starting to add compounds to provide a healthier appeal. A few examples include calcium fortified orange juice for bone health, plant sterols added to foods for cholesterol and blood lipid reduction, and added fiber for heart and digestive health.

Public demand for less processed and preserved foods is on the increase. Case in point is the boom in organic foods. The appeal of organic foods is they are grown without synthetic chemicals and are not subject to hormonal or chemical alteration. Many consumers are willing to pay more for these and other foods with less processing, additives and preservatives.

The food industry is responding. More companies are developing products with fewer additives and preservatives. Many restaurant chains are also hearing the cry of the consumer. While the supersize portion remains alive and well, smaller portion sizes are becoming available on restaurant menus. A few options that restaurants now offer include grilled or broiled versus fried; instead of French fries, alternatives such as fresh fruit, sliced tomatoes, and steamed vegetables are now offered. Opting for dressings and sauces on the side is now a choice we all can make. We still, however, have a long way to go as far as improving our nutrition and food intake. It will take more demand on the part of the consumer to make healthier foods, food products, and menu choices a permanent fixture in our food supply.

When it comes to the environment, a number of manufacturers are starting to "get it" and are changing their ways. Many have become more particular about where their product ingredients come from and how they are brought to market. They look at the practices of agriculture, marine stewardship, and other environmental and societal factors. Additional considerations include use

---

Nutrition Note: Some foods tend to have higher pesticide residue levels. A few of these include apples, bell peppers, celery, cherries, imported grapes, nectarines, peaches, pears, potatoes, red raspberries, spinach and strawberries. Therefore, it is suggested that purchasing the organic option may be of benefit to reduce potential pesticide exposure.

Additionally, if produce with the skin or any type of leafy green is on the menu, organic may be the safer product to purchase. Some fruits and vegetables with fewer pesticide residue levels include asparagus, avocado, bananas, broccoli, cauliflower, sweet corn, kiwi, mango, onions, papaya, peas and pineapple.[6]

of natural resources in packaging and transportation. These areas are going to continue to become a critical part of the business environment and shape not only available resources, but economics on a global scale.

New Science

Nutritional Genomics

Scientists are continually finding evidence of how our bodies are designed by our genetics. Each of us possesses our own unique DNA. It's what makes up our genetic blueprint. The study of human genetics continues to reveal just how unique each individual is in their genetic make-up. Another exciting outcome of nutrition research and science is the study of nutritional genomics, which includes *nutrigenomics,* and *nutrigenetics.* According to Ruth DeBusk, Ph.D., R.D., co-author of *It's Not Just Your Genes!* (BKDR Publishing), "… Nutrigenomics is about the individual's environment acting on the genes, and nutrigenetics is about genes acting on the individual's environment, which include nutrition and lifestyle."[7] The research on this subject is looking at methods to "… define the best match between our food choices and our genetic makeup, providing a solid foundation upon which to base diet-related disease interventions and health promotion approaches … dietary components, as functional foods or dietary supplements, will be used to increase or decrease the expression of particular genes to improve health."[8]

Our genes both interact with and react to what we put into our bodies. Food is one of a number of environmental factors that plays a part in this process. This new science is expected to ultimately allow us to match our genetic makeup and the types of food and lifestyle choices that will keep us healthiest. It is similar to tests that have been around for different types of hyperlipidemia (elevated blood fat levels), diabetes, and cancer(s).

Nutritional genomics is a relatively new science, so stay tuned for more information. A few websites for additional information include *www.gdx.net* and *www.ilgenetics.com*. If you do have yourself tested and results show you may benefit with nutrition and lifestyle intervention, consult your healthcare practitioner and a registered dietitian for assistance. In 2008, the Genetic Information Nondiscrimination Act (GINA) was passed. This Act "… will protect Americans against discrimination based on their genetic information when it comes to health insurance and employment… and will pave the way for people to take full advantage of the promise of personalized medicine without fear of discrimination."[9] For more information, go to *www.genome.gov/27026050.*

Nanotechnology

Another exciting development on the horizon is nanotechnology. The United States National Nanotechnology Initiative (NNI) defines nanotechnology as the understanding and control of matter at dimensions between 1 and 100 nanometers.[10] A nanometer (nm) is defined as one billionth of a meter.[11-14] To put it in perspective, a nanometer is ten thousand times smaller than a strand of human hair; a sheet of paper is approximately 100,000 nanometers thick; and an inch is 25,400,000 nanometers.[15]

Nanotechnology utilizes materials from 1-100 nm in size.[16] While some materials have a known function or property, they can be manipulated through nanotechnology to develop a different and more useful function.[17] So what does this have to do with food, nutrition, and health? Quite a bit.

In the food industry, packaging products are being developed to detect and prevent spoilage of foods contaminated with organisms such as Escherichia coli (E. coli) and other harmful pathogens. An example of one such product is an edible nanolaminate that can prevent oxidation and spoilage of foods; it is under experimentation.

Another example is an antibacterial nanomist that can detect the growth of harmful organisms on produce and kill them at the time of harvest.[18,19]

In the area of nutrition, products made with nano-vehicles are in the works. Nano-vehicles could provide a delivery system to enhance the absorption of some nutrients that are not easily metabolized by the body, such as some vitamins, minerals, antioxidants, and phytonutrients. One example is vitamin D. Vitamin D is a fat soluble vitamin, and is difficult to incorporate in lowfat or nonfat dairy products. The use of a nano-vehicle may improve the bioavailability and solubility of the vitamin in the food product.[20]

As consumer interest in functional foods expands, the potential for nanotechnology is immense. The creation of nanoemulsions, nanofibers, nanofilms, nanocomposites—the list goes on—to improve nutrient absorption, along with food safety will continue to be researched.

In medicine, another huge potential exists. Alternatives in the detection and treatment of conditions such as Type 1 diabetes, wound healing, cancer, atherosclerotic plaque buildup, and other conditions are on the forefront with this technology. Individuals have the potential to be treated on a case-by-case basis versus a one-size-fits-all approach.[21-24]

Other areas of nanotechnology include its use in sports equipment, cosmetics, electronics, solar energy, water desalination, and environmental benefits.[25,26]

This is a relatively new science and more research on initial and long term effects and safety to the body and environment need to be acquired, reviewed and approved before implementation. For more information, go to *www.nano.gov, www.nsf.gov/news/news_ summ.jsp?cntn_id=100602* and *www.nano.gov/html/facts/whatIs Nano.html.*

Chapter 2

Buyer Be Aware

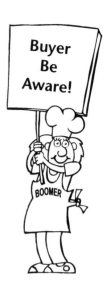

Never Underestimate the Power of Advertising

The majority of us boomers can say we have all been influenced in one way or another by some type of media and advertising. The technology of our times lends itself as an easy vehicle to promote products or services day and night. Advertising is a powerful and profitable component of business. It is designed to create a need and get you to buy what is being sold. With the use of slick audio and visual effects used today, it is no wonder that our brains are stimulated, and thus our impulses are as well. The theory of effective marketing is repetition. The belief is if you hear and see it enough, you may feel you actually need this product and are persuaded to buy it. Think about the tropical vacation ads in the middle of winter—they work!

Another hook is presenting the commonality of an ailment or situation. Presenting the average person who has been transformed into a vibrant, attractive and healthy individual by a particular product is just irresistible. Think of how many commercials in which we have heard or seen that example repetitively. After a while, we end up humming the tune to many of them, along with associating the tune to the product. It also doesn't hurt to have an attractive model promoting it either.

With all of the broadcasting now available via the television alone, there are more channels than ever devoted exclusively to selling products. A new product of our times is the infomercial industry. It too is huge and profit oriented. These programs are scripted and rehearsed just like a television show. While there are many credible products and services being presented, there are also many that the consumer should think about before buying. Interviews with alleged experts—interviews that tell you how wonderful their breakthrough is—have been rehearsed many times over. Often, these experts will tease but not tell you just what the "breakthrough" is without your investment in the product. You then find out after purchasing the product that it really isn't so spectacular after all. If you are going to invest in a product for your health, you owe it to yourself to be sure it's legitimate. Some of the websites you can use to research new products are: *www.healthfinder.gov, www.consumer.gov, www.nccam.nih.gov, www.ods.od.nih.gov, www.ftc.gov/health*, and *www.cfsan.fda.gov*.

Also look for the seal of Infomercial Testimonial Group (they independently test products and solicit real testimonials from consumers) on a company's website, or the television screen. Request a sample. If a monthly commitment is required, look elsewhere.

Here's something to note about the 30-day guarantee. Many times your package will take three weeks to arrive. In actuality, therefore, you have one week to try it out. Many products require a few weeks of use before results can be noted. Ask about this before placing an order.[1]

The Promise of Eternal Youth

Aging is not an easy process. It happens to all of us at some point or another. Some of us are blessed with better genetics than others. We have no idea what is in store until the process begins. Hormonal changes, lack of sleep, arthritis, memory loss and the like, are just a few of the symptoms associated with the aging process. One of the trends these days is the promise of more energy, better sex drive, looking younger, and whatever else the charlatan is peddling.

One of the products out there purporting to make us young is Human Growth Hormone (known as HGH, HcG or others like it). HGH is considered a drug, just like any other prescription medication. Some people are getting these injections from individuals who are not qualified medical professionals. There has not been enough concrete evidence to show these products are safe and long lasting. Messing with hormones is a dangerous thing. Keep in mind that there are documented studies showing some cancers are hormone mediated.

There have been a number of large and credible studies looking at hormone replacement therapy in women and whether it reduced the risk of cancer and heart disease. It showed that there was mixed evidence as far as any benefit.[2] For some, hormone replacement therapy has helped alleviate hot flashes and slow osteoporosis. However, hot flashes eventually go away and there are now medications and supplements to treat osteoporosis.

Reality hits us all at some point. If you feel you need some help with hormonal changes you may be experiencing, consider consulting an endocrinologist (a physician who specializes in treating the endocrine system). A formally trained and legitimately credentialed healthcare professional, such as a registered dietitian (RD), can help counsel and coach you in nutrition and metabolism. It's important to ask about credentialing because your life and health are worth a few questions. You wouldn't go to a car mechanic to get your computer repaired, would you?

While it is not easy to contend with emotionally or physically, aging is a natural process of life. The best proven remedies for making us feel better and move a little easier are exercise and good nutrition—something that is accessible, not ridiculously expensive and a whole lot safer. Some of the websites listed in the previous section and throughout this book can help provide suggestions in regards to finding a credible practitioner and appropriate questions to ask.

Detoxification

We hear and read about detoxification products and processes quite often. While we do live in an environment that contains a number of contaminants, there has yet to be any real product (aka advertised via infomercial/print media) that has been scientifically proven by the mainstream medical community to detoxify our bodies. We have a liver, digestive system and kidneys that absorb the necessary nutrients from what we consume and discard what is not needed. Skin is our largest organ, and perspiration rids our bodies of waste as well.

"Cleansing" is a fad that comes and goes. The theory behind using a cleansing agent is to purge the body of toxins. Some products are taken orally, or some individuals use enemas or colonic treatments. The majority of these products work by irritating the intestines, which is similar to what laxatives do. Many of them can potentially be harmful if used on a regular basis. When taking some of these products, side effects can include diarrhea, nausea, and an upset in electrolyte and fluid balance, which, in some exceptional cases, can even be fatal. The colonic procedure can also result in diarrhea, nausea, cramps, fluid and electrolyte imbalance. On occasion an abdominal puncture can occur with this procedure, thus leading to infection and other complications.

The medical community has mixed reactions on the use of these types of treatments. There are some supplements and regimens that qualified healthcare practitioners will recommend for individuals with certain needs, such as someone exposed to toxic materials, to assist in ridding toxins, thus "detoxifying" the body.

These individuals are closely monitored when such a regimen is prescribed. Consuming plain water, engaging in some exercise, and eating a high fiber diet with fruits, vegetables and whole grains is really the easier and more reliable remedy for most people to keep their digestive system working well. Most of these products are made with compounds from them anyway, so why not enjoy the pleasure of eating them?

If you are interested in discussing foods and supplements that support your immune system discuss this with a qualified healthcare practitioner vs. an advertisement. There are too many individual factors for a one-size-fits-all product. Throughout this book we review strategies to boost your health through good nutrition and lifestyle.

It's all about consistency. Our bodies are designed to rid themselves of waste on a *daily* basis, not once or twice a year. Investing in an expensive product is probably not going to provide any added benefit.

Simply increasing our fiber intake and ridding our bodies of excess waste can give us a great energy boost, especially if we have sluggish digestion. So when you hear about all this extra energy people have due to elimination and cleansing, think fluids and fiber versus pills and potions. Also, think get moving (exercise) to increase blood flow, circulation and digestion.

Some individuals cannot tolerate certain types of fibers. Before beginning any such regimen, discuss this with your physician or healthcare practitioner.

Increase fiber gradually so that your body can adapt and adjust. The addition of products such as bran should also include increasing your fluid intake to prevent potential gas, bloating, and constipation.

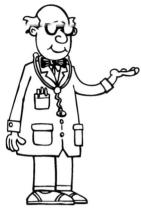

Types of Medicine and Those Who Practice It

A lot of people want and need health education. These days, it can be confusing deciding who to turn to for credible information and counseling. While initials after a person's name don't mean everything, they do stand for something. It is important to ask about the experience and education behind those initials when making a choice in your healthcare.

Registered Dietitian

Many folks are unfamiliar with the difference between a **Registered Dietitian** (RD), a **Nutritionist**, and other titles people claim or possess. In the United States, to become an RD, an individual must attend an accredited college or university, receive a bachelor's degree and complete course work approved by the American Dietetic Association (ADA). They also must complete a supervised and accredited internship (1200 hours), pass a national examination, and complete continuing education requirements to maintain registration (75 continuing professional education units/CPEUs over a five year period). Some states also require an RD to have a license.

Many RDs call themselves nutritionists, but a nutritionist cannot claim the RD title. RDs can also specialize and receive board certification in many different areas of nutrition. A few areas include sports medicine, gerontology, renal, pediatrics, and oncology. Additionally, many join practice groups with specific areas of interest, such as integrative and functional medicine (alternative therapies), sports and cardiovascular nutrition, food and culinary, business and industry, physical medicine and rehabilitation, HIV/AIDS, school nutrition, vegetarianism, and many more.[3] To find nutrition information and an RD in your area, visit the website for ADA at *www.eatright.org*.

Dietetic Technician, Registered

A **Dietetic Technician, Registered (DTR)**, works in the many areas of food and nutrition as well. Depending on the environment they work in (such as nutritional counseling), DTRs work under the supervision of, or in partnership with RDs. In other areas, they work independently, such as food service administration.

Education requirements consist of a minimum of an associate degree obtained from an accredited institution along with 450 hours of supervised practical experience through an accredited dietetic technician program, pass a national examination, and maintain registration status through continuing education (50 CPEUs over a five-year period). A DTR may fulfill requirements by obtaining a baccalaureate degree concurrent with fulfilling the didactic program in dietetics criteria which has been established by the Commission on Dietetic Registration of the ADA. When going this route, a DTR must also pass a national examination and maintain registration status through continuing education.[4] For more information, go to *www.eatright.org*.

Nutritionist

A **Nutritionist** title can take on many definitions. Some nutritionists may have many years of credible education and experience, however, some may have received a certificate from attending a curriculum of a few months with little or no supervised experience. Let's take a look at a few different types of nutritionists:

> A **Certified Nutritionist (CN)**® attends a distance learning program which is administered by the Huntington College of Health Science (*www.hchs.edu*). The institution is accredited by the Accredited

17

Commission of Distance Education and Training Council (*www.detc.org*). The program consists of six courses, a 150 hour internship and a comprehensive final examination administered by American Health Science University (*www.ahsu.edu*) and the National Institute of Nutritional Education (NINE). To maintain a CN® an individual must complete 16 contact hours or two continuing education units (CEUs) per year.[5]

The Certification Board for Nutrition Specialists defines a nutritionist as a health specialist focusing their profession on the use of food and nutrition in the prevention and treatment of a number of diseases and nutrition related deficiencies. The organization was founded in 1993 by the American College of Nutrition (ACN).

To become a **Certified Nutrition Specialist (CNS)** an advanced degree (such as a master's or doctorate) is required. As with an RD, successful completion of a written examination along with relevant documented clinical experience is necessary to acquire a CNS certification. The ACN also has continuing education criteria for maintaining the CNS status.[6] The website for the Certification Board for Nutrition Specialists is *www.cbns.org*.

A **Certified Clinical Nutritionist (CCN)** fulfills criteria established by the Clinical Nutrition Certification Board. This includes an examination and recertification every five years, along with completing an established scope of practical experience in clinical nutrition.[7] For more information regarding CCNs go to *www. cncb.org*.

As nutrition is often an elective in most medical schools, very few physicians are well educated in nutrition. The **Physician Nutrition Specialist®** (PNS) generally has a background in some type of medicine and/or subspecialty. Individuals complete defined nutrition training along with satisfying the requirements of the American Board of Physician Nutrition Specialists (ABPNS).[8] The website for ABPNS is *www.main.uab.edu/Sites/abpns*.

Chiropractic Healthcare

Chiropractic Healthcare places an emphasis on the body's musculoskeletal structure (primarily the spine) and function. While treatment functions do vary, **chiropractors** perform spinal and other body part adjustments to help restore alignment and help the body heal itself. They may also prescribe and perform other therapies including rehabilitative exercises, electrical stimulation, and nutrition counseling, to name a few.

In the United States, it is necessary for a practitioner to earn their Doctor of Chiropractic (D.C.) from an institution accredited by the Council on Chiropractic Education (CCE). For those interested in attending a chiropractic college, applicants must have approximately two to four years of undergraduate coursework with an emphasis on the sciences. Training is typically a four-year academic program encompassing classroom and practical experience in patient care. Additional training may be acquired for those who wish to specialize. Continuing education is required to maintain credentialing.[9] For more information, check out *www.acatoday.org/*.

Chiropractic care is considered part of complementary and alternative medicine (CAM). CAM is a group of diverse medical and healthcare systems, practices, and products that are not presently considered to be part of conventional medicine.[10] Conventional medicine is medicine practiced by holders of M.D. (medical doctor) or D.O. (doctor of osteopathy) degrees and by other allied health professionals, such as physical therapists, psychologists, and registered nurses.

There are healthcare practitioners who practice both CAM and conventional medicine. While some scientific evidence exists regarding some CAM therapies, there are still questions yet to be answered. These questions include whether these therapies are safe and whether they work for the conditions for which they are used. CAM therapies are continually changing as is healthcare treatment. Many people have turned to using CAM for their health.

Complementary and alternative medicines are different from each other. Complementary medicine is used in conjunction with conventional medicine. One example is using aromatherapy to alleviate discomfort.

Alternative medicine is used in place of conventional medicine. An example is using a special diet to treat an illness instead of conventional medicine. Integrative medicine is a combination of conventional, complementary and alternative medicine. The National Center for Complementary and Alternative Medicine (NCCAM) is the Federal Government's lead agency for scientific research on CAM. Its mission is to explore complementary and alternative healing practices in the context of rigorous science, train CAM researchers, and disseminate authoritative information to the public and professionals.[11] The website for NCCAM is *www.nccam.nih.gov.*

Practitioners of Naturopathy

In the United States, professionals who practice naturopathy generally fall into one of several groups:

Naturopathic Physicians

They are educated and trained in a four-year, graduate level program at one of the four U.S. naturopathic medical schools accredited by the Council on

Naturopathic Medical Education (*www.cnme.org/*). Admission requirements include a bachelor's degree and standard premedical courses. The study program includes basic sciences, naturopathic therapies and techniques, diagnostic techniques and tests, specialty courses, clinical sciences, and clinical training. Graduates receive the N.D. (Doctor of Naturopathic Medicine). Postdoctoral training is not required, but graduates may pursue it. Depending on where they wish to practice, naturopathic physicians may also need to be licensed. The scope of practice varies by state and jurisdiction. For example, some states allow naturopathic physicians with special training to prescribe drugs, perform minor surgery, practice acupuncture, and/or assist in childbirth.

Naturopathic physicians are trained to know that herbs and some dietary supplements can potentially interact with drugs, and to avoid those combinations. To do so, they need to be informed of all drugs (whether prescription or over-the-counter) and supplements that you are taking.[12]

Conventional Practitioners with Naturopathic Training
This group consists of licensed conventional medical practitioners (such as doctors of medicine, doctors of osteopathy, dentists, and nurses) who pursue additional training in naturopathic treatments, and possibly other holistic therapies. Education and training programs for this purpose also vary.[13]

Side Effects and Risks
Naturopathy appears to be a generally safe healthcare approach, especially if used as complementary (rather

than alternative) medicine, but several qualifying points are important:

- Naturopathy is not a complete substitute for conventional medical care.
- Some therapies used in naturopathy have the potential to be harmful if not used properly or under the direction of a trained practitioner. For example, herbs can cause side effects on their own and interact with prescription or over-the-counter medicines. Restrictive or other unconventional diets can be unsafe for some people.
- Some practitioners of naturopathy do not recommend using some or even all of the childhood vaccinations that are standard practice in conventional medicine.
- The education and training of practitioners of naturopathy vary widely.

Some Other Points to Consider
Tell your healthcare practitioner about any complementary and alternative practices you engage in. Give them a full picture of what you do to manage your health. This will help ensure coordinated and safe care.
Talk to the practitioner about:

- His/Her education and training, and any licensing or certification.
- Any special medical conditions you have and whether the practitioner has had any specialized training or experience in them.[14]

Reprinted with permission from *www.nccam.nih.gov*.

Trainers

Another location where people are exposed to health education is the fitness center or gym. Trainers will work with clients to assist them in improving their physical fitness. Some trainers do have an education in exercise physiology or physical medicine. Many, however, do not have a thorough education in nutrition. Often trainers may be given incentives to sell nutritional supplements (including beverages, energy bars and the like) along with the fitness consultation. These products can be expensive and may not necessarily provide any more benefit than a sensible diet.

In summary, there are a lot of individuals with initials after their name. When seeking any practitioner for nutrition or health advice, ask pertinent questions regarding education and credentialing to protect yourself. There are plenty of folks out there who are informed, but not necessarily educated and credentialed in nutrition or healthcare. Trust your instincts. If someone is trying to sell you something and you don't have a good feeling about it, I suggest you go elsewhere. To further research complementary medicine, supplements, and the like, a great website to start is *www.nccam.nih.gov/*. For information to find an exercise physiologist in your area go to *www.asep.org*; for a physical therapist, go to *www.apta.org*.

Chapter 3

Supplements, Antioxidants and Food Allergies

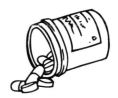

The Case for Supplements

While many strive to eat well, maintaining a daily regimen to supply necessary nutrients can be challenging. Factor in environment, health, aging, medication use, stress, malabsorption, and bioavailability of nutrients, and it is not surprising nutrition deficiencies may prevail. Regular consumption of nutritional supplements can be an adjunct to providing essential vitamins and minerals many may not consume in their daily food intake.

For example, in athletes and aging men, creatine supplements have been shown to improve muscle strength for short duration.[1-3] Omega-3 fatty acid supplements may play a role in a number of conditions including heart health, mood, and arthritis.[4-7] Research continues to explore the roles of compounds in supplement form and their potential benefit in health. Supplementation, however, is not a substitution for healthy eating.

The dietary supplement industry is a multi-billion dollar industry. Consumer spending for supplements nearly doubled from 1994 to 2000, and it continues to grow 10 percent a year.[8,9]

There are factors to consider in regards to supplements. One of the best ways to understand what you may benefit from is to consult a qualified healthcare practitioner who specializes in nutrition and supplementation. Randomly taking supplements based on a news story or print article may be hazardous to your health. As interactions between supplements and medications can occur, it is important for you to review all supplements and medications you are consuming with your healthcare practitioner. Pharmacists are also a great resource for this.

A physical exam along with other tests and a dietary analysis may reveal nutritional deficiencies or a health condition which can assist in recommendation of supplements. Many a practitioner treats conditions such as diabetes, depression, cardiovascular disease, arthritis, etc. with nutritional supplementation.

The variety of nutritional supplements is staggering. A number of supplements are available only through credentialed and licensed practitioners. These particular manufacturers do extensive research and testing of their products to assure quality and adhere to safety standards to protect the consumer. Many also conduct research on their products with credentialed practitioners specializing in research.

While some supplements prove no harm, there are some that are ineffective, potentially dangerous, or marketed using fraudulent claims. Products have been recalled due to microbiological, pesticide, heavy metal contamination or addition of ingredients containing steroids or stimulants. In addition some do not contain the dietary ingredients they are represented to contain; or they contain more or less than the amount of the dietary ingredient claimed on the label. In those cases found, the FDA took enforcement actions and issued warnings due to undeclared ingredients, sub-potency and contamination.[10] Be mindful when claims such as fat burning or energy enhancing are on the label. This could indicate added sugars, caffeine, and other compounds. Check the ingredients and review them with a qualified healthcare practitioner.

In order to ensure consumers' access to legitimate dietary supplements the 1994 Congress passed the Dietary Supplement Health and Education Act (DSHEA). This act provided the FDA the authority to protect the public against supplements that pose safety concerns or mislead the consumer. Under this act, a dietary supplement manufacturer must ensure that its products are safe and that statements about them are not false or misleading.[11]

The FDA itself does not analyze dietary supplements before they are sold to consumers. The manufacturer is responsible for ensuring that the "Supplement Facts" label and ingredient list are accurate, that the dietary ingredients are safe, and that the content matches the amount declared on the label.

By law, a manufacturer may make three types of claims for their dietary supplement product: health claims, structure/function claims, and nutrient content claims. These are not medical claims. Some supplements have a wording or disclaimer that states "This statement has not been evaluated by the FDA. This product is not intended to diagnose, treat, cure or prevent any disease."[12] This statement is required by law. The manufacturer is responsible for ensuring the accuracy and truthfulness of these claims and is therefore required to state a disclaimer.

Claims to treat, mitigate, cure or diagnose any known illness, injury, disease or disorder are medical claims. Only a drug can legally make such a claim. Products such as powders, liquids and bars are considered food unless they claim to be a dietary supplement; they are then required to provide a supplement fact panel on their product.[13]

The supplement fact panel will provide the following:

- An appropriate serving size
- Information on 14 nutrients, when present at significant levels including sodium, vitamin A, vitamin C, calcium and iron and other vitamins and minerals if

they are added or are part of a nutritional claim on the label
- Dietary ingredients for which no Dietary Reference Intakes (DRI) have been established
- If the product contains a proprietary blend of ingredients, the total amount of the blend (although amounts of individual ingredients in the blend are not required).[14]

The rule requires that the labels of products containing botanical ingredients identify the part of the plant used to make products. The source of the dietary ingredient may either follow the name or be listed in the ingredient statement below the "Supplement Facts" panel. When the terms "high potency" or "antioxidant" are used on a food label, the following applies:

- **High Potency** may be used to describe a nutrient when it is present in a food product including dietary supplements, at 100 percent or more of the DRI established for that vitamin or mineral. The term may also be used with multi-ingredient products if two-thirds of the nutrients that are in the product are present at levels that are more than 100 percent of the DRI.
- **"Antioxidant"** may be used in conjunction with currently defined claims for "good source" and "high" to describe a nutrient where scientific evidence shows that following absorption of a sufficient quantity, the nutrient will inactivate free radicals or prevent free radical initiated chemical reactions in the body.[15,16]

The FDA issued its final rule establishing regulations to require current good manufacturing practices (CGMPs) for dietary supplements. The final CGMPs became effective June 2008 for large companies; companies with less than 500 employees had until June 2009; companies with fewer than 20 employees had until June 2010 to comply with the regulations. The goal of these practices is to ensure manufacturers produce unadulterated and properly labeled supplements. A few of these practices include:

- Requirement that proper controls are in place for dietary supplements so they are processed in a consistent manner and meet quality standards.
- These practices apply to all domestic and foreign companies that manufacture, package, label, or hold dietary supplements, including those involved with testing, quality control, packaging, labeling, and distributing them in the United States.
- Consistency in manufacturing as to identity, purity, strength and composition.
- Requirements including provision related to design and construction of physical plants that facilitate maintenance, cleaning, proper manufacturing operations, quality control procedures, testing final product or incoming and in-process materials, handling consumer complaints, and maintaining records.

The FDA does make cyclical inspections to dietary supplement manufacturing facilities. If any type of violation is found or if corrective action is needed, the manufacturer is required to provide evidence that they have rectified the situation.[17]

However, even with this legislation there are challenges. A 2010 report published in Consumer Reports in collaboration with Natural Medicines Comprehensive Database (NMCD) revealed that only one-third of the 54,000 dietary supplements in the NMCD exhibited some component of safety or effectiveness backed by scientific evidence.[18] Along with this, supplement manufacturers are not required to demonstrate safety or efficacy of their products when introducing them to the market.[19]

While no system is perfect, CGMPs are a first step in developing guidelines for supplement manufacturers to adhere to. Let's hope this is the beginning of more effective and stringent standards that will be put into place for the protection of the consumer.

When shopping for a supplement, look for manufacturer contact information. Look for products that have a USP or NSF/ANSI 173 on their label. Either of these symbols indicates that the product has been tested for content, contaminants, and that the product has been manufactured according to CGMPs established by the FDA. U.S. Pharmacopeia (USP) is an official public standards authority for all prescription and over-the-counter medicines and other healthcare products sold or manufactured in the United States. National Sanitation Foundation (NSF) is an independent not-for-profit organization committed to protecting the public by certifying products, and writing standards for food, water, and consumer goods. American National Standards Institute (ANSI) is a private nonprofit membership organization that coordinates development and use of voluntary consensus standards and conformity assessment systems.

Finding these symbols on supplements can be challenging. Many supplement manufacturers utilize third parties for purity certification. For more information, go to *www.usp.org, www.nsf.org*, or *www.ansi.org*.

If you experience any type of reaction to a dietary supplement you can either contact your healthcare practitioner, the product manufacturer, or FDA Medwatch *www.fda.gov/medwatch/how.htm*.

Can Supplements Help Extend Life?

Researchers are examining the consistent consumption of nutritional supplements and the role they may play in health and life extension. A few studies have examined what supplementation does to telomere length, which can be a window to the aging of a cell.

What's a telomere? A telomere is likened to a bookend on the end of a chromosome (a long strand of DNA). Telomeres play a role in cell division and protect the chromosome from fusing or binding with other DNA. Each time a cell divides, a telomere will shorten. If the telomere becomes too short, DNA damage may occur. In some cases, this process may be linked to cancer, where certain cells will stop replicating while others continue to grow. Some scientists will measure the age of a cell by the length of its telomere. The shorter the telomere, the less likely it will continue to replicate, indicating a somewhat "aged" telomere. Telomeres are also susceptible to oxidative stress. Antioxidants play a role in combating the effects of oxidation.[20]

In a study of 586 women (ages 35 to 74), consistent use of multivitamins was associated with longer telomeres (~5.1 percent). Consumption of foods containing higher levels of vitamins C and E also showed an increase in telomere length.[21]

Another study looked at the effect of green tea on telomere length. Tea contains polyphenols, which are a group of anti-oxidants. Green tea has a polyphenol content of from 30 to 40 percent, while black tea has from 3 to 10 percent. This particular study evaluated 976 Chinese men and 1,030 Chinese women over 65. The higher amount of green tea consumed (about three cups per day in this study), the longer the telomere length.[22]

Nutrition Note: Some medicines and herbs can interfere with or counteract each other, which can affect your health. Be sure to discuss with your healthcare practitioner.

A study performed at the University of California, San Francisco, looked at the effect of omega-3 fatty acids and telomere length. Six hundred eight individuals with stable coronary artery disease participated. Telomere length was measured at baseline and at five years. Those individuals who consumed omega-3 fatty acids EPA (eicosapentaenoic acid) and DHA (docosahexaenoic acid) experienced a slower rate of telomere shortening. Omega-3 fatty acids have been linked with anti-inflammatory properties, thus potentially reducing oxidative stress.[23] DHA has been associated with brain and eye health, while EPA plus DHA have been linked with cardiovascular and other health conditions.[24]

Some researchers have noted that those individuals who consume supplements may have a healthier lifestyle overall. These are a small sample of studies performed on the relationship of multivitamins and antioxidants in relation to health and aging. For more conclusive and specific evidence, additional study data is necessary. In the meantime, evaluating the use of supplements and consuming green tea is something to discuss with your healthcare practitioner.

The Importance of Vitamin D

Once thought to be associated only with bone conditions, the role vitamin D plays in overall health and immunity has expanded in recent years. Research is revealing that the role this vitamin may play in health is extensive. This includes:

- Cancer
- Cardiovascular disease
- Rheumatoid arthritis
- Diabetes
- Irritable Bowel Syndrome
- Immunity
- Chronic Liver Disease

- Muscle Weakness
- Multiple Sclerosis
- Metabolic Syndrome
- Neuromuscular Function
- Mood Elevation
- Infectious Diseases[25-42]

Function of Vitamin D

The primary role of vitamin D is the regulation of calcium and phosphorus allocation into the bones.[43] Without adequate vitamin D, bones can become brittle, thin, or misshapen.[44] Vitamin D deficiency can occur at any stage in life; in children a deficiency can cause rickets; in adults the potential for osteopenia or osteoporosis.[45-47]

Sources and Variables

Vitamin D possesses unique attributes. One of four fat soluble vitamins, it is converted to a steroid hormone by the body. It is the only vitamin our bodies manufacture through the synthesis of sunlight exposure.[48-50]

There are two forms of vitamin D: vitamin D_2 (ergocalciferol) and vitamin D_3 (cholecalciferol). D_2 is derived from plant and yeast sources while D_3 is synthesized from sunlight and also derived from animal sources.[51-53] Because it is able to withstand temperature variations and is more stable due to one less double bond, D_3 is utilized more often in food processing.[54]

There has been some question as to which form of vitamin D is more potent. Firm conclusions regarding different effects between the two have not been reached; it does appear, however, at higher doses D_2 is less potent.[55,56] Stay tuned for more updates.

The National Osteoporosis Foundation recommends a daily intake of 400 to 800 IU (International Units) for adults under 50, and for those over 50: 800 to 1,000 IU.[57]

The best food sources include fatty fish, such as salmon, tuna, and fish liver oils. Additional sources include beef liver, egg yolks, and cheese. Vitamin D in these foods is primarily in the form of D_3 and its metabolite $25(OH)D_3$.[58-61] Mushrooms with enhanced levels of vitamin D_2 from exposure to ultraviolet light under controlled conditions are under experimentation.[62-64] Much of the vitamin D in the American diet is consumed through fortified foods. Some examples of vitamin D fortified foods in the United States include milk, ready-to-eat cereals, juices, yogurt, and margarine.[65-68] The table on the next page lists some sources of vitamin D. Both vitamin D_2 and D_3 are available in supplement form. Many calcium supplements also contain vitamin D.

In addition to food and supplements, the "sunshine vitamin" D is produced endogenously when ultraviolet rays (UVB) from sunlight strike the skin and stimulate vitamin D synthesis.[69,70] When exposed to summer sunlight for 20 to 30 minutes, the skin will produce ~10,000 IU of vitamin D.[71] Some studies suggest that 5 to 30 minutes of skin exposed to sunlight (without sunscreen) between 10 a.m. and 3 p.m., at least twice a week, is adequate for vitamin D synthesis.[72-74]

A large number of people can therefore meet their daily vitamin D needs through sunlight exposure. However, as we age, our bodies synthesize vitamin D at a slower rate. For example, when a 70 year old and 20 year old are exposed to the same amount of sunlight, the 70 year old makes ~25 percent of the vitamin D_3 the 20 year old is able to make.[75]

Vitamin D synthesis can be affected by a number of factors. These include season, geographic latitude, time of day, cloud cover, smog, shade, skin melanin content, and pollution.[76-79] These variables can reduce UV energy by 50 to 60 percent. Vitamin D synthesis does not occur with exposure to indoor sunlight through a window; UVB radiation does not penetrate through glass.[80,81]

Selected Food Sources of Vitamin D

Food	IUs per serving*	Percent DV**
Cod liver oil, 1 tablespoon	1,360	340
Salmon (sockeye), cooked, 3 ounces	794	199
Mackerel, cooked, 3 ounces	388	97
Tuna fish, canned in water, drained, 3 ounces	154	39
Milk, nonfat, reduced fat, and whole, vitamin D-fortified, 1 cup	115-124	29-31
Orange juice fortified with vitamin D, 1 cup (check product labels, as amount of added vitamin D varies)	100	25
Yogurt, fortified with 20% of the DV for vitamin D, 6 ounces (more heavily fortified yogurts provide more of the DV)	80	20
Margarine, fortified, 1 tablespoon	60	15
Sardines, canned in oil, drained, 2 sardines	46	12
Liver, beef, cooked, 3.5 ounces	46	12
Ready-to-eat cereal, fortified with 10% of the DV for vitamin D, 0.75-1 cup (more heavily fortified cereals might provide more of the DV)	40	10
Egg, 1 whole (vitamin D is found in yolk)	25	6
Cheese, Swiss, 1 ounce	6	2

*IUs = International Units.

**DV = Daily Value. DVs were developed by the U.S. Food and Drug Administration to help consumers compare the nutrient contents of products within the context of a total diet. The DV for vitamin D is 400 IU for adults and children age 4 and older. Food labels, however, are not required to list vitamin D content unless a food has been fortified with this nutrient. Foods providing 20% or more of the DV are considered to be high sources of a nutrient.

The U.S. Department of Agriculture's Nutrient Database Website, *http://www.nal.usda.gov/ fnic/foodcomp/search*, lists the nutrient content of many foods and provides a list of foods containing vitamin D: *http://www.ars.usda.gov/SP2UserFiles/Place/12354500/Data/SR22/ nutrlist/sr22a324.pdf*. A growing number of foods are being analyzed for vitamin D content. Simpler and faster methods to measure vitamin D in foods are needed, as are food standard reference materials with certified values for vitamin D to ensure accurate measurements.

Source: *www.ods.od.nih.gov/factsheets/VitaminD_asp.*

The moderate use of commercial tanning beds that emit 2 to 6 percent UVB radiation is also effective in stimulating vitamin D synthesis.[82,83]

Vitamin D producing rays can be blocked with the application of sunscreen. Sunscreens absorb both UVA and UVB radiation prior to it entering the skin. The ability of the skin to absorb and produce vitamin D_3 can be impaired by up to 95 percent with a sunscreen containing sun protection factor (SPF) of 8 and up to 98 percent with a sunscreen containing SPF 15 if used properly.[84] Most people, however typically do not apply adequate amounts, nor do they reapply it regularly when outdoors.[85]

Increased skin pigment reduces the capacity of skin to synthesize vitamin D_3. Those individuals with darker skin have a higher melanin content; melanin acts like a natural sunscreen, tending to absorb more of the UVB rays when sunlight strikes the skin. Therefore an individual with higher melanin content may need longer exposure to the sun.[86,87]

While the exposure to sunlight is important for vitamin D synthesis, it is important to emphasize the incidence of skin cancer associated with long term UV radiation from the sun as well as the potential from commercial tanning beds. UV radiation is a known carcinogen and is responsible for the majority of skin cancer and metastatic melanoma cases in the United States. Other cosmetic skin changes have been associated with long-term UV exposure, such as dryness and premature aging.[88-90]

Special Considerations

As vitamin D is a fat soluble vitamin, some dietary fat is required for absorption. Individuals suffering from fat malabsorption (such as in the case of cystic fibrosis, liver disease, and Crohn's disease) may benefit with supplementation.[91-93] Obesity (BMI > 30) can alter the release of vitamin D into circulation due to excess fat, as well as leading to a lower plasma concentration.[94] Gastric bypass patients may need additional supplementation because the area of the upper intestines, where vitamin D is absorbed, is "bypassed."[95,96]

Testing for Vitamin D

The best indicator of vitamin D status is serum concentrations of 25(OH)D. This concentration reflects vitamin D produced cutaneously (through the skin), as well as that consumed from diet and supplements.[97] This serum concentration has a circulating half life of two to three weeks.[98,99] As vitamin D is fat soluble, any excess is stored in body fat and the liver. Circulating $25(OH)_2D$ is generally not a good indicator of vitamin D status because it has a short half life of 15 hours, and levels typically don't decrease until vitamin D deficiency is severe.[100,101]

Discussion remains over optimum serum concentrations of 25(OH)D in relation to overall health. The table on page 38 refers to current established levels and their relevant health status.

Excessive Vitamin D and Medication Interaction

While vitamin D toxicity is not common, it is possible to consume excessive amounts of vitamin D in supplement form. Vitamin D toxicity can cause a variety of symptoms, some of which include nausea, vomiting, poor appetite and weakness.[102] Excessive levels of vitamin D can also cause calcium levels to rise, which can lead to heart rhythm changes and mental confusion.[103] Results from the Women's Health Initiative revealed that over a seven year period, postmenopausal women who consumed daily supplements of 1,000 milligrams of calcium and 400 IUs of vitamin D had a 17 percent increase in the incidence of kidney stones.[104] If you have a history or family history of kidney stones this is something to discuss with your healthcare practitioner.

Serum 25-Hydroxyvltamln D [25(OH)D] Concentrations and Health*

nmol/L**	ng/mL*	Health status
<30	<12	Associated with vitamin D deficiency, leading to rickets in infants and children and osteomalacia in adults
30–50	12–20	Generally considered inadequate for bone and overall health in healthy individuals
≥50	≥20	Generally considered adequate for bone and overall health in healthy individuals
>125	>50	Emerging evidence links potential adverse effects to such high levels, particularly >150 nmol/L (>60 ng/mL)

*Serum concentrations of 25(OH)D are reported in both nanomoles per liter (nmol/L) and nanograms per milliliter (ng/mL).

**1 nmol/L = 0.4 ng/mL

Source: Office of Dietary Supplements, National Institutes of Health.
http://ods.od.nih.gov/factsheets/VitaminD_pf.asp.

In regards to supplementation, the Institute of Medicine (IOM) suggests a safe upper limit of 4,000 IU per day for most adults.[105] Anyone taking steroids, cholesterol-lowering agents, weight-loss products (such as Xenical© and Alli™), and anti-seizure medications should discuss vitamin D with their healthcare practitioner as these agents can interfere with absorption.[106-108]

The Future of Vitamin D

Research is revealing some exciting data about the role vitamin D plays in our health. Imagine if a number of the conditions mentioned can be improved (or at least reduced in severity) by simply increasing vitamin D intake. Stay tuned, as more data is sure to be forthcoming.

Prebiotics, Probiotics and Immunity

We've been hearing more about live cultures called *prebiotics* and *probiotics*. What are they?

Prebiotics are compounds that stimulate the growth of healthy bacteria in the intestines. They are naturally occurring, but can also be synthesized.[109,110] Fibers, starches and sugar alcohols are a few examples.[111] More examples are shown in the accompanying chart.

Probiotics are small, live organisms that help sustain the health of our intestines. Some of the more common are Lactobacillus and Bifidobacteria, both found in yogurt and other fermented dairy products, such as kefir and buttermilk (be sure to check the label for live active cultures).[112-114] The majority of foods with probiotics are refrigerated, because the cultures are destroyed through heating.

According to the International Food Information Council Foundation, "Probiotic bacteria taken together with prebiotics that support their growth are called 'synbiotic.' Both work together in a synergistic way to more efficiently promoting the probiotics' benefits."[115] Typically, probiotics are used to assist in:

- Reducing symptoms of bloating and diarrhea from lactose intolerance
- Diarrhea from antibiotics
- Diarrhea in infants (with rotavirus enteritis)

There is the potential that probiotics can assist in boosting our immunity and intestinal health, alleviate irritable bowel syndrome, and decrease the risk of certain cancers and high cholesterol levels.[116-119]

Probiotics can also be found in supplements. While their exact efficacy is not known, some people use them in pill, powder, or liquid form. More research and experimentation with probiotics is sure to come.

Listed in the following table are a few sources of Prebiotics and Probiotics:

Examples of Probiotics and Prebiotics

Class/Component	Source*	Potential Benefit
Probiotics		
Certain species and strains of Lactobacilli, Bifidobacteria, Yeast	Certain yogurts, other cultured dairy products, and non-dairy applications	May improve gastro-intestinal health and systemic immunity
Prebiotics		
Inulin, Fructo-oligosaccharides (FOS), Polydextrose, Arabinogalactan, Polyols—lactulose, lactitol	Whole grains, onions, bananas, garlic, honey, leeks, artichokes, fortified foods and beverages, dietary supplements and other food applications	May improve gastro-intestinal health; may improve calcium absorption

Chart adapted from International Food Information Council Foundation: *Media Guide on Food Safety and Nutrition: 2004-2006.*

*Examples are not an all-inclusive list.

Reprinted with permission from International Food Information Council Foundation *www.foodinsight.org/Resources/Detail.aspx?topic=Functional_Foods_Fact_Sheet_ Probiotics_and_Prebiotics.*

Following are some recipes utilizing yogurt, which is a great source of probiotics. Yogurt also makes a great substitute for sour cream or mayonnaise in some recipes.

For those of you who stop by your local coffee shop for what I call a loaded beverage, try substituting the following recipe. It can save you time, money, and is more nutritious than coffee with milk, sugar and syrup. It will also give you more sustained energy and not put you on the sugar caffeine roller coaster. Make it ahead of time and take with you to work.

Recipes

Recipe Acronyms: PRO = protein,
CHO = carbohydrate, FAT = fat, Chol = cholesterol

Mocha Banana Split Smoothie

1/2 cup 2% milk

1 cup plain nonfat yogurt

1 banana, cut into pieces

1 Tbsp. unsweetened cocoa powder

2 Tbsp. natural peanut butter

1-2 tsp. instant coffee crystals, depending on preference of strength

2 Tbsp. ground flaxseed

1-2 cups crushed ice, depending on preferred consistency

Mix all ingredients in food processor or blender.

For some added decadence, top with some shaved dark chocolate or chocolate covered espresso beans. Makes 2 servings.

Per serving (without chocolate): 260 calories, 16 gm PRO, 27 gm CHO, 10 gm FAT, 7 mg Chol, 7 gm Fiber, 332 mg Calcium, 154 mg Sodium, 798 mg Potassium

Yogurt Sour Cream Cheese Dip

2 cups plain nonfat yogurt, drained

1/2 cup salsa, drained

1 cup light/reduced fat sour cream

1 cup frozen chopped spinach, thawed

1/2 eight-ounce can, water chestnuts, chopped (use remainder in a tossed salad or soup)

Place yogurt and salsa in a colander/sieve and allow to drain at least 60 minutes. Ideally, allowing yogurt to drain in the refrigerator will keep it at optimum and safe temperature.

Discard liquid.

In medium bowl mix yogurt, sour cream, spinach, water chestnuts, and salsa.

Place a cover over bowl, refrigerate and allow flavors to blend for 2-3 hours.

Serve with vegetables, crackers, or use a spread on wraps and sandwiches. 9 servings.

Per serving: 73 Calories, 4 gm PRO, 7 gm CHO, 3 gm FAT, 10 mg Chol, 1 gm Fiber, 150 mg Calcium, 99 mg Sodium, 270 mg Potassium.

Antioxidants

Many conditions and diseases are brought on by inflammatory responses. According to Andrew Weil, M.D., "We used to think there was a different trigger for each condition (heart disease, cancer, Alzheimer's), but research is pointing to more and more out-of-control inflammation as the single thread."[120] Some of the responses are due to a reactive process in the body from what we consume.

In the digestive process molecules known as free radicals are produced when foods are broken down. Other environmental factors such as tobacco, ultraviolet light, and radiation can cause them to form as well. Free radicals are unstable molecules that can damage cells, tissue, and DNA.[121] Free radicals can cause oxidation and over time, their damage may play a role in contributing to poor health. Antioxidants are compounds that can help counteract the effects of free radicals.[122]

Let's break the word down: *anti* is against and *oxidation* is when a food or chemical changes and tends to breaks down. An example is when you cut into an apple or pear. In a short time, it begins to brown. That's oxidation. If you mix it with some citrus juice, that prevents it from browning—that's an antioxidant in action. Antioxidants are compounds found in foods, such as vitamins A, C, E, some minerals including selenium, copper, zinc, and compounds such as carotenoids, flavonoids, lycopene, and polyphenols.[123,124] They can be looked on as a nutritional ally in immune function. Think:

antioxidant =
anti-inflammatory + more nutrition

Many of the same compounds can combat different health conditions. Numerous studies have shown the benefit of antioxidants in risk reduction in a variety of conditions including:

- age related macular degeneration of the eyes
- heart disease
- asthma
- certain cancers[125,126]

An easy way to select foods with antioxidant properties in most cases is to think of foods with deep color. A few examples of these include:

- **Red**—Red Peppers, Strawberries, Tomatoes, Watermelon, Raspberries, Apples, Cherries, Pomegranate
- **Orange**—Oranges, Sweet Potatoes, Apricots, Cantaloupe, Carrots, Peaches, Winter Squash, Mango, Persimmons, Clementines

- **Yellow**—Grapefruit, Turmeric, Lemon, Pineapple
- **Green**—Spinach, Kale, Turnips, Collards, Broccoli, Celery, Green Peppers, Kiwi, Cabbage, Green Tea, Celery, Bok Choy
- **Blue**—Blueberries, Grapes
- **Violet**—Acai, Blackberries, Eggplant, Plums, Dried Plums/Prunes
- **Brown**—Coffee, Black Tea, Unsweetened Cocoa Powder, Mushrooms

Additional food sources and compounds they contain can be found in the **Examples of Functional Components Table** in this chapter.

Nutrition Note: The better source of antioxidants is eating the actual food itself. Many compounds cannot be replicated in pill form. While dietary supplements do exist and can possibly provide benefit, there is more research to be performed regarding their efficacy for certain health conditions.[127] In some cases, dietary supplements can actually aggravate rather than assist in treating certain conditions. This is why it is essential to consult a qualified healthcare practitioner or a pharmacist who can assist you in your particular needs.

Don't Forget the Herbs and Spices

For those of you a bit hesitant to increase fruits and vegetables, heads up. Antioxidant compounds can be found in herbs and spices as well. For example:

- Parsley contains vitamins A, C and K, and also contains beta carotene.[128,129]

- Thyme contains flavones, which may play a protective role in inflammation.[130,131]
- Rosemary has been used to treat a variety of ailments, a few of which include improving memory, relief of muscle pain, and stimulation of the nervous and circulatory systems.[132,133]
- Chives contain vitamins A, C, and K.[134]
- Cilantro is loaded with beta carotene, lutein, zeaxanthin, quercetin, and vitamin K.[135,136]
- Turmeric has been associated with improving mental status.[137,138]
- Cinnamon has been shown to play a role in lowering blood sugar (thus helping diabetics), along with decreasing cholesterol and lowering blood pressure (cardiovascular disease). As little as a quarter teaspoon per day of cinnamon (larger doses may be harmful) can have such an impact.[139-141]
- Oregano has lots to offer, including vitamins, minerals, phytochemicals and the carotenoids lutein, zeaxanthin, and beta-carotene. It also contains compounds that have been linked with potential cancer risk reduction, along with antimicrobial properties.[142]
- Ginger is a source of powerful antioxidants. It has been shown to reduce symptoms of conditions ranging from arthritis, nausea, heart disease, Alzheimer's, and it has been found to slow cancer growth in animals.[143]

Keep in mind we are all in the learning stages of many of these compounds. Researchers are experimenting with dosages, impacts, etc. If we start using these compounds once in a while instead of or in addition to salt and pepper, it will add more taste to our foods, and may actually be of benefit in the long run. Be aware that some of the compounds suggested in *Boomer Be Well* may have an effect on medicines you are currently taking; they may also interfere with a health condition or upcoming surgical procedure. Discuss this with your healthcare practitioner or a pharmacist. Another website to refer to possible herb/supplement medication interactions is *www.nlm.nih.gov/medlineplus/druginfo/herb_All.html*.

A great read to help you understand which foods are an ally in your health is *101 Foods That Could Save Your Life*, by David Grotto, RD, LDN (Bantam Dell). It is an A to Z guide describing the history, nutrition and "how to" prepare or incorporate foods for optimum nutrition.

Changes That Occur When Cooking Food

There are also new findings about how we prepare our foods. Cooking foods at high temperatures for a period of time changes their molecular structure. For example, when starchy foods such as potato and cereal products are cooked at a high temperature for a period of time (such as in potato chips and French fries) the starch undergoes a chemical transformation. A compound called acrylamide is formed. Acrylamide has been shown to cause cancer in animals.[144,145] The possible affect on human health in unclear.[146] On the positive side, there is research being performed to test compounds that may stop the chemical reaction that causes acrylamide to form.[147]

A similar transformation occurs in muscle proteins (beef, lamb, game meats, poultry, pork, and fish) that are grilled at high temperatures. Compounds called heterocyclic amines (HCAs) are formed when the amino acid creatinine is broken down during high heat cooking. HCAs have been shown to be carcinogenic in animals. Additionally, meats that are cured or smoked also increase exposure to cancer-causing agents. A suggestion would be to reduce exposure to these foods. In regards to cooking, either partially pre-cook the meats and then place them on the grill to cook them until done, or cook at lower temperatures and avoid eating the burnt pieces. Steaming, poaching, stewing, boiling and braising are all example of lower heat methods of cooking.[148-151]

Another easy alternative is right in your spice cabinet. Herbs and spices contain powerful antioxidant compounds which may counter the effects of oxidation. Some of the top antioxidant seasonings include cloves, turmeric, ginger, cinnamon, oregano, rosemary and basil.[152-154] Additionally, vinegar or citrus juice such as lemon, lime or orange can help to tenderize proteins. Use canola oil in marinades when cooking proteins at high temperatures. Canola oil has a higher smoking point than olive oil which can reduce smoking or burning. When making a marinade, reserve some in a separate dish to use after cooking for a final basting. Each of the following blends is based on mixing with one pound of protein. They can be used to mix in burgers, marinades or rubs. Here are a few blends to consider:

Blends

Recipe Acronyms: PRO = protein,
CHO = carbohydrate, FAT = fat, Chol = cholesterol

Herbal Blend:

1 tsp. each rosemary, oregano, and basil

2 Tbsp. minced dried onion

1/2 tsp. garlic powder

Per Tablespoon: 12 calories, 0 gm PRO, 3 gm CHO, 0 gm FAT, 0 mg Chol, 1 gm Fiber, 1 mg Sodium

Spice Blend

2 tsp. cinnamon

1 tsp. ginger

1/4 tsp. ground cloves

Per teaspoon: 15 calories, 0 gm PRO, 4 gm CHO, 0 gm FAT, 0 mg Chol, 3 gm Fiber, 2 mg Sodium

Rub/Marinade Blend

1/2 tsp. salt

1 tsp black pepper

1/2 tsp. ground cloves

1 tsp. oregano

1 tsp. turmeric

1/2 tsp. chili powder

Per teaspoon: 4 calories, 0 gm PRO, 1 gm CHO, 0 gm FAT, 0 mg Chol, 1 gm Fiber, 295 mg Sodium

It is up to you what you put in your body. For a healthy individual eating and enjoying barbecued and fried foods in reasonable portions and on an occasional basis should not pose a health risk. Another positive note is that fruits and vegetables don't contain the amino acids that muscle meats do, so they can be grilled guilt free. Overcooking them, however, does reduce the vitamin content.

Nutrition Note

The following table refers to compounds in foods and their potential benefit in certain conditions. It is a great resource.

Examples of Functional Components*

Class/Components	Source*	Potential Benefit
Carotenoids		
Beta-carotene	carrots, various fruits	neutralizes free radicals radicals which may damage cells; bolsters cellular antioxidant defenses
Lutein, Zeaxanthin	kale, collards, spinach, corn, eggs, citrus	may contribute to maintenance of healthy vision
Lycopene	tomatoes and processed tomato products	may contribute to maintenance of prostate health
Flavonoids		
Anthocyanidins	berries, cherries, red grapes	bolster cellular anti-oxidant defenses; may contribute to maintenance of brain function
Flavanols—Catechins, Epicatechins, Procyanidins	tea, cocoa, chocolate, apples, grapes	may contribute to maintenance of heart health
Flavanones	citrus foods	neutralize free radicals which may damage cells; bolster cellular antioxidant defenses
Flavonols	onions, apples, tea, broccoli	neutralize free radicals which may damage cells; bolster cellular antioxidant defenses
Proanthocyanidins	cranberries, cocoa, apples, strawberries, grapes, wine, peanuts, cinnamon	may contribute to maintenance of of urinary tract health and heart health

Examples of Functional Components*

Class/Components	Source*	Potential Benefit
Isothiocyanates		
Sulforaphane	cauliflower, broccoli, Brussels sprouts, cabbage, kale, horseradish	may enhance detoxification of undesirable compounds and bolster cellular antioxidant defenses
Phenols		
Caffeic acid, Ferulic acid	apples, pears, citrus fruits, some vegetables	may bolster cellular antioxidant defenses; may contribute to maintenance of healthy vision and heart health
Sulfides/Thiols		
Diallyl sulfide, Allyl methyl trisulfide	garlic, onions, leeks, scallions	may enhance detoxification of undesirable compounds; may contribute to maintenance of heart health and healthy immune function
Dithiolthiones	cruciferous vegetables— broccoli, cabbage, bok choy, collards	contribute to maintenance of healthy immune function
Whole Grains		
Whole grains	cereal grains	may reduce risk of coronary heart disease and cancer; may contribute to reduced risk of diabetes

Chart adapted from International Food Information Council Foundation: Media Guide on Food Safety and Nutrition: 2004-2006.

*Not a representation of all sources.

For more information on additional beneficial components of food, visit Background on Functional Foods.

Examples of Antioxidant Vitamins and Minerals

Vitamins	Daily Reference Intakes*	Antioxidant Activity	Sources
Vitamin A	300-900 µg/d	Protects cells from free radicals	Liver, dairy products, fish
Vitamin C	15-90 mg/d	Protects cells from free radicals	Bell peppers, citrus fruits
Vitamin E	6-15 mg/d	Protects cells from free radicals, helps with immune function and DNA repair	Oils, fortified cereals, sunflower seeds, mixed nuts
Selenium	20-55 µg/d	Helps prevent cellular damage from free radicals	Brazil nuts, meats, tuna, plant foods

Chart adapted from Food and Nutrition Board Institute of Medicine DRI reports and National Institutes of Health Office of Dietary Supplements.

*DRI's provided are a range for Americans ages 2-70.

For information on Daily Reference Intakes for specific populations go to: *www.iom.edu*.

Food Allergies, Intolerances and Sensitivities

Each year, millions of people have allergic reactions to food. Some can cause minor symptoms, while others can be more severe.[155] Some people may develop:

- Tickle, itch or burning in the mouth or back of the throat
- Headache
- Body Aches
- Nausea, vomiting, diarrhea
- Abdominal cramps
- Hives
- Flushed skin
- Swelling in the face, lips, tongue, throat or vocal chords

- Coughing/wheezing
- Dizziness/light-headedness
- Difficulty breathing
- Loss of consciousness

When a person with food allergies ingests a food allergen, a life-threatening reaction called anaphylaxis can occur. This can lead to:

- Constricted airways in the lungs
- Severe lowering of blood pressure and shock (also known as anaphylactic shock)
- Suffocation by swelling of the throat

Each year in the United States, it is estimated that anaphylaxis to food results in:

- 30,000 emergency room visits
- 2,000 hospitalizations
- 150 deaths[156]

Prompt administration of epinephrine by an autoinjector, such as Epi-pen, during early symptoms of anaphylaxis may help prevent these serious consequences.

_____

Source: www.fda.gov/Food/ResourcesForYou/Consumers/ucm079311.htm

---

A food allergy is the body's reaction to a protein (allergen) in a particular food that triggers an immune response.[157] Food allergy and allergic disease include a number of different conditions that can be categorized as either immunoglobulin E (IgE) or non-IgE mediated.[158] IgE is a protein molecule that acts as an antibody.[159]

Both IgE and non-IgE involve the immune system.[160] The IgE response is usually quick. It can occur within minutes or up to an hour after ingesting an allergen. A non-IgE mediated response is slower and may take hours to days to become evident, as it often manifests in the gastrointestinal tract.[161]

Food allergies are a growing concern. Differences in diagnosis and treatment have existed for quite some time. Some conditions such as food intolerance (which are non-allergenic) can be confused with food allergy.

Because there is a need for a consistent set of definitions and diagnostics, the National Institute of Allergy and Infectious Diseases (NIAID), part of the National Institutes of Health, collaborated with more than 30 professional organizations, federal agencies, and patient advocacy groups, to create a set of guidelines for the diagnosis and management of food allergy. They were issued in 2010.[162] The recommendations emphasize the need for an individualized approach to diagnosis and treatment. To be accurate, diagnosis of food allergy must include *all* of the points below:

- Detailed medical history
- Physical examination
- Diet diary
- Elimination diet
- Skin test
- Blood test
- Oral food challenge[163,164]

As there is no current cure for food allergies, treatment of symptoms and avoidance of the allergen is the best route to follow.[165,166] Wearing an alert bracelet is also a good idea. Washing hands frequently and reading food labels is important.

The Food Allergen Labeling and Consumer Protection Act of 2004 was passed to help Americans avoid the health risks associated with food allergens. The law applies to all foods regulated by the FDA, both domestic and imported. The FDA regulates all foods except meat, poultry, certain egg products and most alcoholic beverages that are labeled on or after January 1, 2006.[167]

There are more than 160 foods that can cause allergic reactions. With the new act, food labels are required to clearly identify the source of all ingredients that are or are derived from the eight most common food allergens, as they account for 90 percent of food allergic reactions. Many food ingredients are derived from these top allergens.[168] These include:

- Milk
- Eggs
- Fish (bass, flounder, cod)
- Crustacean shellfish (shrimp, crab, lobster)
- Tree nuts (pecans, almonds, walnuts)
- Peanuts
- Wheat
- Soybeans

Source: *www.fda.gov/Food/ResourcesForYou/Consumers/ucm079311.htm*

When reading a label, the name of the food source of a major allergen must appear:

- In parentheses following the name of the ingredient such as Lecithin (soy), flour (wheat), whey (milk)
                              OR
- Immediately after or next to the list of ingredients in a "contains" statement, such as "Contains wheat, milk, and soy"

Some labels will also state the product was manufactured in a facility that processes allergens, such as "Made in facility that processes nuts, wheat, etc."[169]

The National Institute of Allergies and Infectious Diseases (*www.niaid.nih.gov*) (NIAID) conducts research on food allergy and other allergic diseases. Several treatment approaches are currently being tested in research settings. These include Immunotherapy with allergen injections, immunotherapy with allergen under the tongue and anti-IgE therapy.[170]

Food Intolerances

In some cases, individuals may not have a food allergy but food intolerance or sensitivity. These tend to be more prevalent than food allergies.[171] A food intolerance is likened to an enzyme deficiency. It is not an immune reaction.[172] One example is wheat intolerance (not to be confused with celiac disease, which is an autoimmune disease—see Chapter 8); another is lactose intolerance, which affects over 75 percent of the worldwide population.[173,174]

Food Sensitivities

Food sensitivities are a common cause of many chronic conditions and affect an estimated 15-20% of the population. Symptoms provoked by food sensitivities occur when our immune system begins perceiving foods in the same way it perceives things which are truly harmful, such as bacteria, viruses, parasites, etc.

There are many reasons why this can happen, but this mistaken identity leads to the release of toxic chemicals called "mediators" (such as histamine, cytokines, and prostaglandins) from our immune cells. It's the inflammatory and pain-inducing effects of the mediators that give rise to symptoms, which ends up making us feel sick. Examples include headache, body ache, nausea, brain fog, and gastrointestinal distress to name a few.[175,176]

According to Jan Patenaude, RD, director of medical nutrition at Signet Diagnostics, "Research has shown that patients with irritable bowel syndrome (IBS), migraine headaches, fibromyalgia, chronic depression, and many other conditions have higher than normal levels of these mediators circulating throughout their bodies." For many, the "trigger" that causes the mediators to be released can be linked to foods or chemicals in their diet.[177]

Food sensitivity symptoms are often chronic because the mediators that make us feel sick are released every time reactive foods or chemicals are consumed. There are tests available to assist in determining food sensitivity. One is Antigen Leukocyte Cellular Antibody Test (ALCAT), administered by Cell Science Systems.[178,179] A newer test is the Mediator Release Test (MRT) administered by Signet Diagnostics.[180-184]

The ALCAT test measures size changes in white blood cells after exposure to various foods, food additives, colorings, environmental chemicals, pharmacoactive agents, and molds.

Food test panels range from 50 to 200 different foods. There are optional tests for additional agents. Test results are revealed on a color coded panel.[184,185] Results should be reviewed with a qualified healthcare practitioner, such as a registered dietitian (RD). If an individual tests positive, a customized program should be implemented with medical supervision. A rotation diet is usually suggested for those tested with ALCAT.[186,187]

MRT is a patented blood test which precisely measures volumetric changes in white blood cells after exposure to foods and chemicals. The most comprehensive MRT test panel includes 150 foods and chemical substances. Dietary modifications based on the testing are best implemented by a Certified Lifestyle Eating and Performance (LEAP) Therapist (CLT). A CLT has undergone advanced training in managing food sensitivities, and has established expertise in understanding the LEAP dietary protocols. The CLT reviews results and then a customized dietary program based on test results is implemented to assist in eliminating the offending food/agent.[188-191] Many people find a relief in symptoms within a short period of time.

> **Nutrition Note:** An interesting note with food sensitivities is that while many individuals strive to consume anti-inflammatory foods and compounds, they may actually have a sensitivity to them.[192] Working with an RD, especially one trained in this area, can help sort it out.

With the increase in food allergies and sensitivities, more people are turning to fresh and unprocessed foods. They are also purchasing more natural types of cleaning compounds for personal and home use.

For additional information on this subject go to *www.niaid. nih.gov, www.aafa.org, www.cspinet.org/* (go to food safety*) www. eatright.org* (go to find a registered dietitian), *www.foodallergy.org.*

For more information regarding sensitivity testing go to *www.alcat.com* or *www.nowleap.com.*

Chapter 4

Food

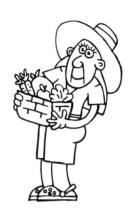

A Trip to the Market

Ever get to the market knowing what you are going to buy and then when you walk in the store your mind just goes blank? With an overwhelming number of products to choose from it is difficult to understand how to shop.

Even before we get to the market we've been bombarded with information (both true and false), advertising (both true and false) and just plain temptation (opinions from the angel on one shoulder and the devil on the other!). Then when we get there it can look like a colorful scene from the Wizard of Oz. We think, okay, this time it's going to be all healthy foods and no junk. All good and no bad. Many a consumer wonders if there really are good or bad foods.

In regards to the "bad" foods, there are foods which are more processed and have ingredients added to them that may complicate a health condition. For example, foods with added sugars can potentially elevate an individual's blood sugar (glucose) levels. For a diabetic or an individual with impaired glucose metabolism, this is something that is important to manage. Other foods have higher levels of sodium than others. For someone with high blood pressure or kidney problems, a high sodium intake may lead to fluid retention, thus potentially increasing blood pressure and putting more work on the heart.

Other additives in foods, such as gluten, can wreak havoc on an individual with celiac disease. Sulfites, monosodium glutamate (MSG), nuts, soy, dairy and other additives can create an allergic reaction in those sensitive to those products. If a product has a long list of ingredients that you just can't understand, look for the fresh or unprocessed alternative. They may have a shorter shelf life, but your health is worth it.

One exception is those products that have been fortified with added vitamins, minerals and antioxidants. For example, a breakfast cereal may be fortified with vitamins and minerals. If the product has a reasonable amount of fortification, then opting to purchase this product may be a good bet if you find supplements too costly. In this way you are getting some added nutrition.

There are a few easy tips to making your trip to the market an efficient one. While this may sound very basic, writing a list prior to going to the store can help keep you focused. Plan your menus ahead of time. Categorize each food group. If you know the layout of the grocery store you frequent, then you know where items are stocked.

For example, if you know you need milk, will you also need butter, yogurt, or cheese? The strategy of shopping the perimeter of the market still holds true. The staples such as produce, meats, dairy, and breads are usually stocked in these areas. The aisles are where the true challenge lies for the consumer in regards to what I will term "temptation" aisles. In addition, the ends of the aisles and the check-out area are designed for a compulsive buy. The packaging on a food product is the selling point. Competition can be fierce. With more interest in nutrition, many food products also contain nutrition/health claims on their labels. Remember that eye appeal is intended to sell, and be sure to read the fine print.

Let's look at some categories of foods that can help save you money and promote good nutrition:

Dairy

Low or nonfat dairy products contain less saturated fat. Even when a food contains no saturated fat, there is a chance that it will contain cholesterol. This has to do with the fact that the structural component of the product contains cholesterol. It is a natural substance in animals (and that includes us primates!).

Look for products without added sugars. You can add your own items for sweetness. For example, plain yogurt can be turned into all kinds of treats. Adding cereal, nuts, dried fruit, fresh fruit, dark chocolate bits, etc., can turn it into a delicious and nutritious meal or snack. If you do buy the sweetened yogurt with the "fruit at the bottom," understand that "fruit" is very close to fruit preserves and has a lot of added sugar.

Produce

Many folks feel that fresh produce is superior to canned and frozen. This is not always the case. Frozen vegetables and fruits are flash frozen and not subject to the conditions of fresh produce such heat, light, air, transportation and time on the shelf. If purchasing frozen produce, look for a product without added sugars, sauces or sodium.

When purchasing fresh produce, look for produce that is not wilted, moldy, pierced or exhibits obvious damage. This could be a sign it has gone bad and has been exposed to contaminants.

If you or your family can only "stomach" vegetables with some type of sauce (kids, this is for you), you can make your own. To make a creamy type sauce, all it takes is a thickening agent such as flour or corn starch, a small amount of fat, such as butter or a plant sterol fortified margarine, and some liquid. Chances are these ingredients are already in your kitchen.

It takes about five minutes to prepare the sauce. You can add your own preferred seasoning, such as herbs, spices, hot sauce, and even cheese. The harder cheeses, such as parmesan, romano, asiago, are more flavorful, so a little goes a long way. When making your own sauce, you know what is in the ingredients.

You can also make other types of sauces for your vegetables. This is a great way to educate your children in cooking with fresh ingredients and take part in the process. There is a greater likelihood that they will consume what they prepare, especially when it comes to vegetables.

Recipe
Recipe Acronyms: PRO = protein,
CHO = carbohydrate, FAT = fat, Chol = cholesterol

Here's an easy white sauce to have on hold:

Simple White Sauce

2 Tbsp. butter or sterol fortified margarine

1-1/2 to 2 Tbsp. flour (rice flour, potato flour or corn starch may be substituted)

1 cup 2% or nonfat milk or a substitute of 1 cup chicken, beef, vegetable or fish stock

(A combination of 1/2 cup milk and 1/2 cup stock may be used.)

In saucepan melt butter/margarine over low heat.

Add flour and mix until well blended.

Slowly stir in milk and/or broth until well blended.

Season to taste with salt and pepper, spices, herbs, grated cheese, etc. Makes 1 cup.

Per Tablespoon (made with 2% milk and butter):
30 calories, 1 gm PRO, 2 gm CHO, 2 gm FAT, 5 mg Chol,
0 gm Fiber, 18 mg Sodium

Canned Foods

Canned foods have come a long way since we were children. Some canned items such as tomatoes, have an increased availability of nutrients, as they are cooked prior to canning. The process of heat can create a release of nutrients and antioxidants, leading to better absorption. Adding a drizzle of some fat can also help with absorption of these compounds. This holds true for some fresh vegetables as well. Lightly steaming carrots, broccoli, and greens, for example, can release compounds that will also assist in better absorption, particularly of antioxidants. When purchasing canned items, look out for the following:

- **Dented or punctured cans**—They may have been subject to damage and contamination.
- **Fruits**—If you are watching your sugar intake, look for fruit packed in water or in its own juice. Fruits with added syrup have added calories via sugar and syrup.
- **Vegetables**—Look for those reduced or low in sodium. Also read the labels for sugars. If there are added sugars, look for those without. If that is not available, you can rinse the product with water and that will reduce the sodium and sugar content.

Grains and Starchy Vegetables

Strive for purchasing products made with whole grains. Some labels indicate if the product is a source of whole grains. Buy products in their unadulterated form. For example a rice blend without seasoning is likely to have very little sodium. Many rice, pasta and potato products with sauces, seasonings and the like do have added sugar and sodium. They may also cost more money. You can season them yourself. Chances are you already have seasoning blends, herbs and spices in your pantry.

If convenience is what you seek, buy the product with reduced cooking time. If you feel you must purchase a "seasoned" product, use a third of the seasoning packet. You will still have the benefit of flavor along with convenience, and consume less salt and other additives.

Be sure to look at the sodium content of blends and rubs. Some can contain quite a bit (over 1000 mg per serving). Recommended daily sodium intake is 1500 to <2300 mg/day. If you are using a blend or rub, you can also extend it with added herbs/spices. Fruit juices and vinegars can make for a great marinade and flavor enhancer on meats, vegetables, and starch dishes. If they are in your pantry, experiment with a few and you may be surprised at what you come up with. There are also many rubs, sauces, and marinades out there that have very few preservatives, salt or sugar added to them. Look for them or ask your grocer.

Protein

There are many options to choose from. Animal products with less saturated fat include lean beef, pork, skinless poultry, low or nonfat dairy products, eggs, fresh, frozen or canned seafood without batter or oil. A variety of vegetarian items made with soy, such as edamame (soybeans), tofu, tempeh and textured vegetable protein are complete sources of protein and make for a great "meatless" meal. Canned beans are also a great source of quality and affordable protein.

Snacks

A trip down the snack aisle is just that. While there is much to choose from, baked items will contain less fat versus fried counterparts. Look at the sugar, fat, fiber, and sodium content of items. We will review this in greater detail in the label reading section. When it comes to dessert items, lowfat or reduced sugar items are now readily available. You can make your own home-made juice pops as well. Popsicle containers are available in stores. Experiment with juice blends. This way you know what is in your food and what you and your family are consuming. Adding items like fresh mint leaves to popsicles or ice cubes can change a flavor profile and make it even more refreshing.

Frozen/Refrigerated Meals

There are many delicious varieties out there. Chances are, many also have quite a bit of sodium. Look for those with around 500 to 700 mg of sodium if possible. Round out the meal with accompaniments such as some veggies, a salad, fruit, and a glass of milk. One interesting point to note regarding individual frozen meals: Portion sizes of the calorie-controlled varieties are something to learn from. They are usually reflective of a recommended serving size, such as a three ounce portion of protein, a serving of carbohydrate and a serving of vegetables.

Buying Meals at the Deli, Grocery or Big Box Stores

In this wonderful age of convenience, sometimes it's just easier to purchase a meal at the grocery store deli. If you are purchasing a combo type meal, and want to buy a side salad or some chips, here are a few ideas:

- If purchasing a mayonnaise based salad (such as tuna, egg, chicken), go for a side salad which has some fresh fruit or vegetables without much (if any) added fat.
- If this particular deli has the best mayonnaise based potato or macaroni salad this side of the Mississippi, swap the protein in the sandwich for straight meat, such

as lean beef or turkey, and get the sandwich dry. This way you can put your own condiments on it, perhaps mustard instead of mayonnaise, or a reduced-fat mayonnaise if your sandwich is just not the same without the mayo spread.

- You can also just ask for the protein, and forgo the bread if you want the starchy salad or some chips. Remember it is important to have some carbohydrates, protein and fat (and fiber if possible) with every meal to sustain blood sugar and keep you humming throughout the day.

Nowadays, grocery and big box stores have more than ever to offer. If cooking is really not your passion, take advantage of the convenience. Keep in mind, many convenience items tend to have a higher sodium content; therefore check the label. We will review strategies throughout this book to help counter this. A few examples for some fresh meals include:

- **Cooked Roasted Chicken**—Buy two or three cooked chickens. Use one for dinner, and accompany it with some fresh/frozen/canned veggies, along with some type of quick-fix carbohydrate such as ready-made mashed potatoes, or quick rice/pasta/grains. As mentioned, home-made is preferable as you know what you are putting in your food. If there is not enough time for it, use convenience for what it is. Instead of reaching for just the salt and pepper, add some herbs or spices (rosemary and garlic, fresh minced or dried ginger, oregano and basil, turmeric). Finish with a salad made from a pre-washed salad mix with some vinegar and a splash of olive oil and perhaps a sprinkle of some grated cheese.

Have a glass of ice cold milk. The remaining chicken can be used for sandwiches, salads, casseroles, tacos, burritos, etc.

- **Soups**—Many grocery stores now have piping hot soup ready to go in the deli; some have ready-to-eat soups in the refrigerated section. Canned or dried soups and entrees are also an option. Look for reduced sodium. Select a soup, grab some freshly baked whole grain bread or rolls in the bakery, add a pre-washed salad (mix up spinach and another salad mixture) with some precut veggies and cherry tomatoes; add some vinegar and a drizzle of olive or canola oil to the salad. Soup is a satisfying, quick energy food. It also can be a great avenue for leftovers. To make it even easier, toss in some veggies when heating up, and there will be one less dish to wash. Have some fresh or frozen fruit with some chopped nuts and dark chocolate chips for dessert.

- **Canned foods**—Canned fish and chicken are easy to use and can whip up a meal in no time. Individual serving cans are also great to have on hand at the office for a meal or midday snack, as well as coming in handy when out with the kids while hiking, at the beach, etc. Pair them up with some fruit, pre-cut vegetables, crackers or bread. Sandwiches, casseroles, spreads are a few more uses with canned fish or meats. The great thing is that they are already cooked and ready to go. Canned beans, vegetables and fruits are also easy to use. Cottage cheese and canned fruit make a great meal or snack.

Food Preparation Tips

To help manage time and meal planning, listed below are a few ideas to streamline time spent in the kitchen.

Recipe

Recipe Acronyms: PRO = protein, CHO = carbohydrate, FAT = fat, Chol = cholesterol

Here's a homemade seasoning blend to try for chili, tacos, casseroles, or used as a rub for roasts. For every pound of meat, use one Tablespoon.

Seasoning Blend

3 Tbsp. paprika

1 Tbsp. turmeric

1/8 tsp. cayenne

1 tsp. garlic powder

2 Tbsp. dried minced onion

1/4 tsp. salt

Per Tablespoon: 44 calories, 2 gm PRO, 8 gm CHO, 1 gm FAT, 0 mg Chol, 3 gm Fiber, 200 mg sodium

Meats

For a roast or ground meat, cook up a large quantity (at least a few pounds) and divide it up into portions for multiple uses, such as:

- Slicing some of the roast for sandwiches
- Freezing some for quick meal prep
- Using some of the meat for making fajitas, stir fry, soups, or stews
- Adding to pasta, rice, grains, mashed or cooked potatoes with added veggies
- Note: You can grind your own meat in a food processor

Recipes

Here are a few recipe suggestions:

Option 1

With ground meat or a roast cut into diced pieces, here's an easy shepherd's pie recipe:

Mix 1 pound of ground meat with your favorite seasoning such as a taco or fajita season packet (again watch the sodium content). Or, try the seasoning blend recipe.

Mix in 1 package frozen veggies such as corn, peas, carrots, lima beans, and spread mashed potatoes mixed with some herbs, such as fresh parsley, cilantro, or rosemary or spices on top.

Option 2

Mix meat with canned tomatoes and some frozen greens, such as spinach, kale or swiss chard. Add some chopped garlic, fresh or dried basil and oregano. Mix with cooked pasta, buckwheat, quinoa or rice.

Option 3

Mini meatloaves or meatballs are great to have available. They make a great make-ahead meal or snack. Make a large batch and freeze in air tight containers. You can top them with everything from tomato/marinara sauce, brown gravy or condiments for a quick meal with added starches and veggies.

Grains/Starchy Vegetables

- Cook up a large batch of rice, pasta, quinoa or millet. Divide into thirds and add some veggies with herbs to one, dried fruit, nuts and cinnamon to another, and keep one plain. Freeze into individual portion size cups or in freezer bags. That way, you've got the starch component of lunch or dinner made and ready to heat up.

- Buy a large quantity of sweet potatoes (orange flesh has the beta carotene) or a large bag of white potatoes and cook them up. Wash and cut into chunks or slices and either steam or bake until they are almost done. If baking, place potatoes on a cookie sheet (to save clean-up time line the sheet with parchment paper or use non-stick cooking spray) and bake in a 425°F oven for about 30 minutes. If steaming, steam for about 20 to 25 minutes. Allow them to cool and then freeze for easy preparation and a satisfying addition to round out a meal. If freezing ahead, add seasoning during the second round of cooking. Use some imagination. For one meal sprinkle some cinnamon and ground ginger on the sweets, and then drizzle with some olive oil and toss. For the white potatoes, chop some fresh garlic and rosemary, a little salt and pepper, and finish with a drizzle of some olive oil. You can also mix the whites and sweets and make a great blend of mashed potatoes.
- For macaroni and cheese, make up a large batch and divide into thirds. Add some spinach, tomatoes and oregano in one; some mixed frozen vegetables with canned tuna and turmeric in another, and keep one plain.

Eating Well on a Budget

There are a number of nutritious foods that are economical. They include:

- Eggs (protein, vitamins, minerals)
- Oatmeal (soluble fiber)
- Canned Beans (protein, vitamins, minerals, soluble and insoluble fiber—the darker the better)

- Grains in bulk such as brown rice, quinoa, millet, pasta
- Bulk Dry Cereal (the less sugar the better)—many of these are fortified with vitamins and minerals—look for them
- Dried Milk (source of protein and calcium)
- Canned Fish (source of protein, omega fatty acids, vitamins and minerals)
- Canned/Frozen Vegetables (preferably with lower sodium or no added salt)
- Frozen or Canned Fruits (in their own juice/no added sugar), Dried Fruits
- Greens, such as turnip, kale, collards, and the like (think dark green, high antioxidants)
- Produce in season and on sale

Buy in bulk, as it can be cheaper. Foods such as berries in the summertime can be frozen and saved for a few months. The same goes for canning, if you have the time.

Here are a few pointers when reading labels. The label should tell you:

- Serving size. **It's important to look at number of servings per container**
- Calories per serving
- Protein
- Fat
- Carbohydrate
- Cholesterol
- Trans-Fat
- Keep in mind, while trans-fats are being reduced and eliminated in foods, that does not mean total fat is being eliminated in that food.

Label Reading

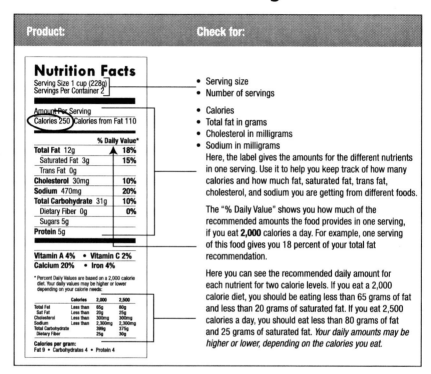

Reprinted with permission from National, Heart Lung and Blood Institute, *www.nhlbi.nih.gov/chd/Tipsheets/readthelabel.htm.*

- Saturated Fat
- Sugars
  - One teaspoon of sugar is 4 gm. Sugar is a carbohydrate at 4 calories per gram. Therefore, 4 x 4 = 16 calories per teaspoon of sugar.
  - Milk has naturally occurring sugars called lactose, so that is why you will see it has sugars listed on a label. Products that have dried fruit added also have naturally occurring sugars as well. Some labels will explain or clarify that and some won't.

- ○ Another way to read for sugar in the ingredients is anything with the last three letters of ose (sucrose, glucose, fructose, etc.).
- ○ High fructose corn syrup is another common added sugar to foods. Others include molasses, invert sugar, corn sweetener, honey and fruit juice concentrate.[1]
- ○ Look for foods that have less than 5 gm sugar per serving. They are out there!
- Sodium (suggested daily intake is <2300 mg/day and for those over 51 or who are African-American or have hypertension, diabetes or chronic kidney disease reduce to 1500 mg/day).[2]
  - ○ Note regarding sodium: Sodium comes in a number of forms—sodium chloride (table salt), sodium bicarbonate, sodium bisulfate, etc. Check the ingredients. If something has >500 to 700 mg per serving, look for an alternative. There are many out there nowadays including soups, frozen meals, etc.
- Listing of some vitamins and minerals
- Fiber
  - ○ Some foods, such as whole grains, seeds, fruits, nuts and vegetables naturally contain fiber. Some have it added (cellulose, pectin). Sometimes fiber is added to help add body and texture to products. Anything with >2 to 3 grams per serving is great!

Ingredients are listed in order by weight. If you are buying a product that claims it is whole grain and the first ingredient is sugar, white flour, etc., look for a product that lists whole grain first. Same goes with fruit juice. You want fruit juice to be the first ingredient versus high fructose corn syrup or sugar. If water is the first ingredient in the product, then that is the ingredient with the higher amount of weight. Get the picture?

Many times sugar and salt are added to foods not only to flavor them, but also to preserve them. Same goes with fats. Over the years, fats became hydrogenated (more hydrogen added to them) to lengthen the product's shelf life and to help keep some foods blended together. A number of food manufacturers are reducing the amount of sugar, salt and fat in their products. Competitor products with fewer additives and processing have created the interest, thus demand for healthier items.

Another note of interest is products that are "sugar free." One way to note this on the label is with a word ending with the letters "ol." For example, xylitol, mannitol, sorbitol. These are sugar alcohols. They are absorbed at a slower rate and thus have less caloric value than a regular, full-fledged carbohydrate. They can also have a laxative effect, which is usually printed on the label, so do keep that in mind if you are trying to watch your sugar intake.[3]

Two sites to refer to for updated nutrition label information are: *www.fda.gov/downloads/Food/LabelingNutrition/Consumer Information/UCM120909.pdf,* along with *www.fda.gov/Food/LabelingNutrition/ConsumerInformation/UCM078889.htm.*

Many grocery store chains have taken on the task of providing nutrition labeling on foods. A number of programs now exist. Program guidelines were created by a panel or individual well versed in the areas of food and nutrition.

A few include Guiding Stars (*www.guidingstars.com*), Healthy Ideas (*www.stopandshop.com*), NUVAL (*www.nuval.com*), Smart Choices Program (*www.smartchoiceprogram.com*), and Smart Tag Program (*www.sfmarkets.com/nutrition/smart-tags*). These programs have been designed to help the consumer in nutrition education when selecting foods.

Safe Food Handling

It seems like food product recalls are occurring on a regular basis these days. Perhaps it is because we have increased communication, or perhaps is due to improved monitoring in our foods. The result of tainted or mishandled food can lead to food contamination and/ or foodborne illness. A few signs of foodborne illness include a headache, body ache, stomach ache or gastrointestinal upset after eating. Many people think they have contracted the flu when actually they are experiencing symptoms of foodborne illness. It can take a few hours and in some cases a day or two to exhibit symptoms.

Nutrition Note: Ever wonder what the difference is between enriched and fortified? **Enriching** a food is putting back what may have been lost in processing. For example, when rice is processed to form white rice, many of the B vitamins and fiber are reduced or lost. Putting those vitamins back is enriching the product. **Fortifying** a product is putting something in that was not originally in the product.[3] For example, calcium fortified orange juice. Oranges do not normally possess much calcium, so fortifying it adds something to the product that was not there. Same goes with a lot of cereals. These products are fortified with vitamins and minerals that were not in the original product.

The Center for Disease Control (CDC) estimates that in the United States foodborne diseases cause approximately 48 million illnesses, 128,000 hospitalizations and 3,000 deaths per year.[4] The Produce Safety Project estimated that in the United States alone, foodborne illnesses cost $152 billion per year. The costs encompass acute foodborne illness and some long-term health related costs.[5]

Many cases go unreported. It is not easy to detect contaminated foods, as they may look and taste safe enough to eat. Those who are at greater risk of exposure to foodborne illness are pregnant women, young children, older persons, and those with a chronic illness or weakened immune system. For these individuals, extra precautions are recommended when consuming any raw or under-cooked meat, pork, poultry, seafood, and eggs, as well as avoiding unpasteurized products such as juices, milk and dairy products, and raw sprouts.[6] While contamination may not be totally pre-ventable, there are strategies we can all utilize to ensure we are doing our best to prevent foodborne illness. Safe and proper handling, preparation and storage can help reduce the likelihood of occurrence. To assist the consumer, many foods such as eggs, meat, poultry, pork and seafood have safe food handling and preparation procedures printed on the package for your safety.

A few additional strategies to keep things clean and safe in your home include:

- Wash hands frequently. Using soap and washing with water that is warm to hot, for 20 seconds (about the time it takes to sing Happy Birthday) can be effective in reducing contamination.
- Always have hand towelettes and/or hand sanitizer on hand for cleaning hands.
- Using soap and hot water or a mild bleach and water solution is recommended for cleaning cutting boards and utensils. Sanitizing products are recommended for counter tops, door knobs, hands and surfaces that do not have direct contact with food.
- After cleaning cutting boards and utensils with hot, soapy water, rinse and allow to air dry. Towels can be a source of contamination if they are not clean. A cleaning/sanitizing solution of 1 Tbsp. unscented bleach to one gallon of water (for a smaller quantity, use 1 tsp. bleach to five cups water) can be used on cutting boards and kitchen surfaces

that will not be damaged by such an agent. Allow the solution to soak for five minutes, rinse with water and allow to air dry. If purchasing another cleaning or sanitizing agent, follow instructions.

- Use separate cutting boards and utensils for produce and animal products. Cross contamination is a common cause for foodborne illness. For example, have one cutting board dedicated to meat, poultry, fish, etc., and one dedicated to produce. Make sure if you are using the same knife, wash it with soap and hot water, and then rinse before using it on other products.

- Pay attention to temperature. Keeping foods at room temperature for more than two hours can start the growth of food pathogens. Refrigerate foods after preparing or purchasing them. Limit the length of time you keep them at room temperature. When having cold foods out at a picnic, try to keep them in a cooler or on ice. A good phrase to remember is "hot foods hot, cold foods cold."

- Keep the refrigerator no higher than 40°F, and keep the freezer at 0°F. Purchase a refrigerator thermometer and place it in the center of the middle shelf. Foods stored on the shelves in the refrigerator door will likely have a higher temperature. Storing perishables such as milk and eggs inside the refrigerator versus on the door may provide for cooler temperatures.[7]

- Clean the refrigerator on a regular basis. Shoot for once a month. Drips, spills, and food fragments can all create bacterial growth. Use a warm soapy solution on shelves, drawers, and doors and then rinse with a clean cloth.

- Many people think mayonnaise is the culprit in salads. The actual culprits are the protein in foods (eggs, chicken, seafood, meats) and human contact. Careful preparation and holding cold salads at a temperature no higher than 40°F can reduce the risk of contamination.[8]

- Wash all skins of produce thoroughly before cutting. When you cut into a product, there is a chance that any surface contaminant can be cut into the flesh of the product. Produce is subjected to the elements of air, soil, temperature, rain, etc., and along with transportation, there is a chance of contamination. Rinsing and drying produce prior to cutting into it can reduce any surface contaminants.
- Any food product that has been subject to human contact has a greater likelihood of becoming contaminated.
- Label and date foods prepared and stored. Practice the rule of first in first out.
- Pay attention to expiration dates on products you are purchasing. Only buy the product if you feel you are going to use it within that timeframe. Dispose of it if it has expired.
- Buy fresh looking produce or products that are not damaged, dented, dirty, moldy or have freezer burn. There is a chance they have already been exposed to some type of contamination if they exhibit any of these signs.
- Use a meat thermometer to indicate the temperature of cooked foods. Typically an internal temperature of 145 to 180°F is desired to assure food is at optimum temperature.[9]

These are only a few tips. A great resource regarding freezing and refrigeration is found in the following tables. They are also available on the website *www.homefoodsafety.org* for a printable version to post in your kitchen. You can also refer to the American Dietetic Association at *www.eatright.org* or your local county health extension for additional information. The website also has additional tips for safe food handling and storage in English and Spanish. Other websites for food safety information include *www.cdc.gov* and *www.foodsafety.gov.*

Refrigerator Calculator

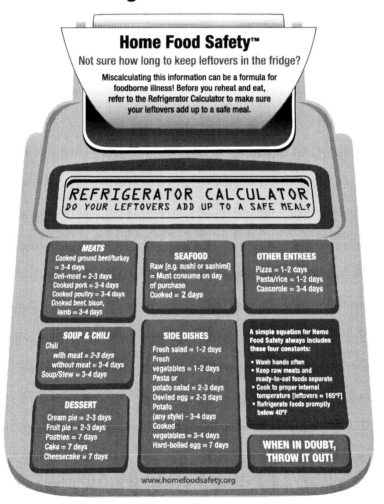

www.homefoodsafety.org/pages/utilities/docs/calculator.pdf.

Reprinted with permission from the American Dietetic Association, 2009.

Keep It Cool:
Refrigerator/Freezer Food Storage Chart

Properly storing foods can help maintain their quality. Make sure perishable foods never sit out of refrigeration for more than two hours, and follow the expiration dates to ensure taste and safety. If no expiration date is available on the package, the following refrigeration guidelines provide a helpful gauge. Freezing is also a smart storage option for shoppers who wish to extend the shelf life of perishable foods beyond their expiration dates. But whether you're freezing or refrigerating, one basic rule applies: When in doubt, throw it out!

Perishable Foods	Refrigerator (below 40°F)	Freezer (at or below 0°F)
Meat (Beef, Pork, Veal, Lamb)		
Steaks	3 to 5 days	6 to 12 months
Chops	3 to 5 days	4 to 6 months
Roasts	3 to 5 days	6 to 9 months
Liver, variety meats	1 to 2 days	3 to 4 months
Cooked meat	3 to 4 days	2 to 3 months
Ground meat		
• uncooked	1 to 2 days	4 months
• cooked	3 to 4 days	
Poultry (Chicken, Turkey)		
Poultry, whole	1 to 2 days	1 year
Poultry, pieces (breasts, thighs, wings)	1 to 2 days	9 months
Giblets	1 to 2 days	3 to 4 months
Cooked poultry	3 to 4 days	4 months
Ground poultry		
• uncooked	1 to 2 days	2 to 3 months
• cooked	3 to 4 days	3 to 4 months
Hot Dogs, Lunch Meat		
Hot dogs		
• opened	1 week	
• unopened	2 weeks	1 to 2 months
Lunch meat		
• opened	3 to 5 days	1 to 2 months
• unopened	2 weeks	
Bacon, Sausage		
Bacon		
• opened	1 week	1 month
• unopened	2 weeks	
Sausage (meat or poultry)		
• raw	1 to 2 days	
• pre-cooked/smoked	1 week	1 to 2 months
Summer sausage (labeled "Keep Refrigerated")		
• opened	3 weeks	1 to 2 months
• unopened	3 months	
Pepperoni, sliced	2 to 3 weeks	1 to 2 months

Keep It Cool:
Refrigerator/Freezer Food Storage Chart

Properly storing foods can help maintain their quality. Make sure perishable foods never sit out of refrigeration for more than two hours, and follow the expiration dates to ensure taste and safety. If no expiration date is available on the package, the following refrigeration guidelines provide a helpful gauge. Freezing is also a smart storage option for shoppers who wish to extend the shelf life of perishable foods beyond their expiration dates. But whether you're freezing or refrigerating, one basic rule applies: When in doubt, throw it out!

Perishable Foods	Refrigerator (below 40°F)	Freezer (at or below 0°F)
Ham, Corned Beef		
Corned beef in pouch with pickling juices	5 to 7 days	Drained, 1 month
Fresh Ham, uncooked		
• uncured	3 to 5 days	6 months
• cured (cook-before-eating)	5 to 7 days	3 to 4 months
	(if dated, follow "use-by" date)	
Ham, fully cooked, store wrapped		
• whole	1 week	
• half	3 to 5 days	
• slices	3 to 4 days	1 to 2 months
Ham, fully cooked, vacuum sealed		
• undated, unopened	2 weeks	
• dated, unopened	Use-by date	1 to 2 months
Ham, canned (labeled "Keep Refrigerated")		
• opened	1 week	1 to 2 months
• unopened	6 to 9 months	Do not freeze
Eggs		
Fresh, in shell	3 to 5 weeks	Do not freeze
Egg whites and yolks (raw)	2 to 4 days	1 year
Egg substitutes		
• opened	3 days	Does not freeze well
• unopened	10 days	1 year
Dairy		
Cheese, hard or processed		
• opened	3 to 4 weeks	6 months
• unopened	6 months	
Cheese, soft	1 week	6 months
Cottage/ricotta cheese	1 week	Do not freeze
Cream cheese	2 weeks	Do not freeze
Butter	1 month	4 months

Note: All recommendations assume refrigerators are set below 40°F and freezers are set to 0°F.

Reprinted with permission from **Home Food Safety™**
www.homefoodsafety.org

Chapter 5
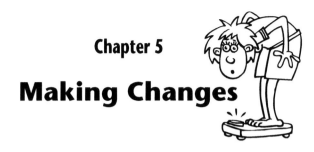
Making Changes

The Dilemma of Dieting

One of the more difficult things about changing patterns and habits in regards to food is that we need to eat. It's part of the body's automatic program of staying alive. We need food because our bodies need nutrients. That's what hunger tells us. "Going on a diet" is similar to taking a vacation. It is a temporary change. When we come back from the "vacation" we go back to our previous routine. Some of us are experts at losing weight. We set the goal of weight loss, go on a diet, and when we reach the desired weight loss, we've accomplished the goal.

Initially, we enjoy how we feel and look, and the compliments people give us are rewarding. We relax and celebrate our success. After a while, old habits return. All of a sudden, the weight has come back, and we are back to going on yet another diet. Thus, the cycle continues. There is always some new type of "diet" popping up or being resurrected. While there are more diets out there than ever imaginable, evidence has shown that the majority of them aren't working. While a number of people may lose weight while on them, over time many gain the weight back and then some.

Michael Dansinger, M.D., of the Tufts-New England Medical Center, and his colleagues looked at results from 46 weight-loss diets totaling nearly 12,000 participants. They reported that the average weight loss was 6 percent, with most dieters regaining all the weight they lost within five years. There was no weight-loss drug or diet that reflected a better result.[1] One reason many diets and weight-loss programs are not long lasting is they don't address individual needs, lifestyle, culture, race, religion, gender, age, food intolerances, etc. What has been shown to be effective is that when people make changes to their lifestyle, they tend to improve their overall health.

One of the keys to success is becoming *conscious*. Successful dieters put the thought and actions into what worked for their individual lifestyle. Many weight-loss packages, programs and pills can be expensive. Some may have lasting results; some do not. Rather than spending the money on yet another expensive program that does not necessarily have statistics going for it, putting the effort into making a few dietary and lifestyle changes based on how you live may end up costing less in the long run. Reducing body weight can reduce risk factors for conditions like heart disease, diabetes, metabolic syndrome and cancer. It also helps us feel better emotionally and physically. Develop your own regimen for *life* and not for the short term.

Thoughts and Beliefs

Many people are under the impression (reinforced by daily media and our society), that you need to be thin to be healthy. However, there are plenty of thin people walking around unaware that they may have such conditions as high blood pressure, elevated blood lipids, or osteoporosis. While maintaining a healthy weight is important, that is not the only factor in wellness.

Before you start applying the principles of this book, visit your healthcare practitioner and get a complete physical exam to give you a baseline of your health. Such an exam should include blood pressure, blood lipids (cholesterol, triglycerides, HDL, LDL, VLDL, etc.), blood sugar, body fat percentage, diabetes, eye health, dental health, and so on. Discuss your intentions with your healthcare practitioner and he or she may have more suggestions for other tests depending on your medical history. Evidence shows that even the slightest increase in physical activity and changes in diet can have significant affects on your health. All you need to do is take the first step. It begins with our thoughts and beliefs.

Our actions are the result of our thoughts. We develop habits and associations of things, and once established we rarely veer from them. We get used to routine. A habit takes time to develop. Changing habits take time as well. On average, it takes three to six months to develop a new behavior. Emotions are also woven into behaviors and reactions. Many of us don't realize how we weave patterns of "protection" into our lives.

For example, some folks use food or cigarettes as a protective barrier between themselves and others. Food/cigarettes become their only friend that never lets them down and is always there for them. But when the weight is lost, or the smoker has quit, the barrier is gone, and so is the friend. Visualizing and planning strategies prior to making any change can be a key to success. Learning how to avoid falling into those old habits is a challenge. The more time you take to make a change or replace a behavior, the more likely it will stay with you for the long term.

There are a lot of success stories out there for people who have improved their quality of life and health. The majority of those folks adapted a new lifestyle their way. They did not deprive themselves, or spend copious amounts of money on pills, potions, and packaging. They ate foods they liked, learned how to incorporate exercise into their lives, and developed a way to deal with stress that was healthy for them. It took time, along with adapting and changing behavior. Those are all positive efforts that can lead to great results.

According to Dr. Dean Ornish, M.D., founder of the Preventive Medicine Research Institute in Sausalito, CA, "People are seeing the connection between what they eat, how healthy they are and how they look and feel…they are realizing that simple changes in their diet can be more powerful than medicine or surgery—not just for living longer but for short term benefits. When you eat healthy foods, your brain, your heart, your skin, and your sexual organs get more blood and nutrients. So you feel more energized, have more sexual potency, look better, and enjoy life more fully."[22] Think of how great you feel and how people see that and tell you so when you're on a roll of taking care of yourself.

Preparing for a Change

Each and every one of us has goals and aspirations for our lives. They are all different. We set them and accomplish them in our own unique way. Most of us have made some changes in our lives that we have been able to adapt and keep. The first thing we did was set a goal. More likely than not, the overall goal was achieved with small behavioral changes. Reflect on how that change came about. Chances are, it took time. Let's say you were able to lose 50 pounds and have kept 20 pounds of it off for the last ten years. You are doing something that is working.

We all know some changes can be tough. While everyone has their own way of accomplishing something, many people have been successful by keeping a journal. Along with keeping a journal, some people write small notes and post them in places to remind them of their goal(s). Before implementing a new pattern keep a journal of your daily activities. Be as specific as you can. Keep a journal of some sort for a few weeks *before* making any change.

The journal could include time of day for all activities such as eating patterns, amount of food eaten, emotions, physical activity and stress load. The overall purpose is to give a realistic reflection of your lifestyle. You may be surprised that simply keeping a journal is an eye opening journey in becoming conscious. Make sure to read and review it on a regular basis.

One key to making long lasting change is to become conscious of what you are doing. Many people are not "aware" when they are eating (along with many other tasks these days). They are pre-occupied with something else, whether it is a conversation, a book, a television show, or a reaction to stress, boredom or some other emotion.

For many, emotional eating is how we have adapted to what I call our *wiring*. We use food as a reactionary device. We plug into it for a response. It's just how some of us have developed our emotional connection.

This connection is not always limited to food. For some it may be cigarettes, alcohol or another outlet. At our stage in life, we are fairly well aware of triggers that can create an emotional chain reaction. A bad day at work, coupled with kids stressed with homework, extracurricular activities that have you doubling as a chauffeur, and a little sleep deprivation can all create for the perfect meltdown.

Sometimes it may seem as our only ally in all the chaos can be found in food. A nice big piece of chocolate cake makes the world a better place. The tricky part about sugar and simple carbohydrates is that they can create a high and low effect on our blood sugar. This reaction can create a "need" for more sugar or simple starches. It is possible to select foods that can actually calm the craving that some foods can create. I suggest eating something with combined protein, carbohydrate, fat and fiber. A few examples of this would be a bowl of cereal or a sandwich. The combination of all three will balance out the blood sugar and should reduce the feeling of being hungry. We will look at other examples throughout *Boomer Be Well!*

Setting a realistic goal is the best way to prepare for a change. More importantly, establishing what you are going to do once you achieve that result is key to your success. Maintenance of the new behavior is the real challenge of creating a new lifestyle. Planning ahead for incorporating new behaviors into your life is part of the success as well. Life includes getting together with friends and family, going on trips (business and pleasure), holidays, and the like. Look forward to adding these new changes. Get friends and family involved as well. If you need additional help in the form of counseling, there are many qualified and trained therapists available.

Writing out your goals and the steps to achieve them is a necessary part of the process. Otherwise, it can be difficult to remember the specifics of your goals. Keep in mind, they are allowed to change. Give yourself options. Some steps may be easy to live with, while others may not work for you. We are all human, thus not perfect, so slips can occur. That is OK. It's also important to write down what has sabotaged you in the past. Refer to your journal so you can reflect on those times when you handled stress better than others.

Write down what you can potentially do for upcoming activities and events. Business meals, snacks in the office, parties, social gatherings, stress and the like are all activities that can catch us off guard. Plan and practice your strategy.

Here's an example: Monday morning meetings at the office always include some doughnuts. Eating one always gets your blood sugar soaring with that cup of coffee. It also makes you hungry a short time later, and then the rest of the day you find yourself reaching for food, and you can't seem to satisfy that hunger. That is one of the effects of simple sugars. Pairing up protein and some fat with simple sugars can help leave you satisfied and not craving for more. There are a few things you can do:

- Eat breakfast at home before the meeting. This way, you may not be as hungry or as likely to reach for that doughnut.

- Offer to bring in the goodies. Bring some bagels or hearty breads accompanied with some lowfat spreads (reduced fat cream cheese, hummus, peanut butter, smoked fish, and the like). You can even ask if something like breakfast burritos might make a nice change. (This way you are getting the combination of protein, carbohydrate, fat and fiber.)
- If you have a cup of regular coffee at home, switch to decaf at the office. Many of us know all too well the caffeine crash we can experience after drinking too much coffee. It can also make us hungry, as caffeine can make our blood sugar levels go up and down.
- Bring in some beverages with the balance of protein, carbohydrate and fat. Examples include lowfat milk, soymilk, yogurt beverages, or even yogurt. Or, just bring in some bottled water.
- Make your own smoothie with the balance of protein, carbohydrate, fat and fiber. To lowfat milk or yogurt you can add fruit, chia seeds, ground flaxseed, wheat germ or bran for fiber. A little fat, such as a nut butter, can help sustain your energy over a longer period of time. Fiber will help blood sugar levels remain steady for a longer period of time as well. Sip on this during the meeting.

This is one example of planning ahead. If you know what may be in store, you are prepared. Also, in this example, everyone is gathered for a meeting not a buffet. If note taking is necessary, offer to do it, as you will be less likely to eat.

Developing New Habits

Based on my personal experience as a nutrition and health counselor, it takes an average of three to six months to adapt to a new habit. Being patient in the process is also a challenge. Often, we wake up one day and decide that we want to lose 20 pounds in a month. Many of us seem to forget that it took a while to gain that weight. In our instant and quick fix society, taking things slowly can seem so difficult. However, life and its events don't all happen at once. We need to remember that life is not about all or none. How boring it would be if it were always the same. No one likes stress that is not pleasant, but it is going to happen.

What may work as a stress alternative in one situation may not work in another. Sometimes you truly can walk away from something and other times you cannot. Learn what diversion can help you cope. For many who lose weight or quit some other habit, the transference of one substance to another is quite common. For example, the relationship we have with the friend such as food, a cigarette or alcohol is likely going to change. Some people cut back on food and use cigarettes as a substitute. The transference develops a new set of habits to contend with. This is why planning ahead and having a variety of options available is so important.

Try different strategies and see what works for you. Talk to people who have made successful changes. Find out how they cope with triggers that come into their life. There are many books, programs and groups available to help in this process. Take advantage of them. The reality is that we all are thrown curve-balls. We react in our own way. Remind yourself that you know how to get back on track and take care of things. It takes conscious thinking and planning.

Think about a situation you were in where you reacted differently and were pleased with how you reacted. For example, maybe you did not turn to food for comfort. Maybe you took a walk, talked with a friend, or hit a round of golf balls instead. It cleared your mind. Life is built on old and new experiences. Many times, the old experiences truly do help us in appreciating the new ones. Trying new things is one of the great things about life. Developing new hobbies can be a lot of fun as well. It's also good for brain health.

Look at making changes in the same way you would starting a new job or learning a new skill. It will take time. We weren't born with specific behaviors; we develop and incorporate them over time. It takes focus and energy to make any change. That's where that passion, patience and persistence comes in—when you are implementing a new pattern and routine. Whatever it takes, you are getting REAL. It's needed for you to succeed.

Our bodies are very forgiving. Think about how they bounce back after childbirth, surgery or an injury. We have to eat, but many times emotions are woven into the event of eating. For example, if you're a stress eater (which many of us are at some point), start thinking about alternatives to food. Try different strategies until you find what works for you.

Another thing we can learn is to trust in ourselves. This is an obstacle for many of us. Often we don't have confidence that we can be successful at making changes. Whether it's personal or professional, many of us think about change, but are hesitant to take that leap. Look in the mirror and say to yourself you can. Understand that life is full of ups and downs. Experience helps shape who you are. We are all working with challenges of some sort. Give yourself credit for your effort. Even when you're in "coast mode" (which is difficult for many of us), enjoy it. It's all in the thought pattern and mindset. You can do whatever you challenge yourself to do and overcome amazing odds.

Maintenance of Behavior

We've looked at a few ways to make some changes. What is even more important is committing to maintain those changes. Some points to consider include:

- **Remember, this is for the long haul.** Take your time and think about the big picture.
- **Give yourself variety with any change you make.** This can avoid boredom and burnout.
- **Food is your ally and does not have to be the enemy.** It's just that we've woven eating with emotions, etc., into our behaviors, responses and the like. This can change.
- **Improving your quality of life is about the internal *and* the external.** Check your external environment. Get rid of any temptations or obvious trigger points that you can. It's the balance of the pyramid of good nutrition, exercise, and stress management that keeps us well. If having sweets, chips, or whatever is a trigger for you, don't tempt yourself by having them around the house. The same thing goes for your work setting. Try having treats you enjoy but have less of an impact on your blood sugar. Pretzels, popcorn, cereal, fruits, string cheese, individual serving treats, and sugarless gum may all be satisfying for you. It is not necessary to have temptations for the children, or in case company drops in. Same goes for quitting smoking. It is not necessary to have them around or subject yourself to a situation that will cause you to "cave" to the craving.
- **Set yourself up for success, not sabotage.** You know that you can make excuses, and that is just what they are. Ask yourself the reason why you are doing what you are doing. Then come up with a commitment and alternative that will make you succeed. You will know when you are ready.
- **Practice ahead of time.** For example, practice learning what actual portion sizes look like on a plate. By doing so, you will have a better way to gauge what is on your plate when dining out.

- **Understand why you are doing what you are doing and pay attention to your actions**. Become conscious. Also pay attention to how your body feels. For example, when you are eating, eat a reasonable bite (not a huge handful), and chew (not inhale) it thoroughly. Enjoy the taste, texture and pleasure of the food you are consuming. It is easy to eat a handful of nuts, candy, or chips without realizing it, let alone even thinking about it. If you are inhaling that bag of M&M's or whatever, try to enjoy each one at a time. This in itself might change a few things.
- **Sometimes when we are stressed, upset—whatever—we reach for food, and we feel better**. Maybe we were hypoglycemic (having low blood sugar) and didn't know it—especially if eating calmed us down. Hypoglycemia can makes us shaky, cranky, spacey, stressed, etc. For people who have hypoglycemia, eating small meals (with that balance of protein, carbohydrates, fat and fiber) throughout the day helps manage blood sugar. Interestingly, many people who have changed their way of eating switch to small frequent meals versus one large meal. They found they have more energy, think more clearly, and just feel better in general. There's also a better chance that if you don't get too hungry you may not be as prone to overeat. One additional note with the noshing throughout the day: It is taking care of your teeth. Be sure to drink water, chew some sugarless gum, or drink some green tea. All have been shown to reduce the acid content left on your teeth after eating.
- **We've all eaten out of boredom or habit**. This is the case particularly in the evenings while watching TV or sitting in front of the computer. For many of us, watching the tube or going online with the computer is our relaxation. While we may not be willing to change those habits

(honestly that's how most of us now live), maybe we can tweak a few things ahead of time. Instead of returning regularly to the kitchen to nibble, plan and prepare a satisfying snack, and then stay away from the kitchen. It's all about planning ahead.

- **When planning meals and snacks start acquiring the mindset of assembling a meal of protein, carbohydrate, fat and fiber.** This strategy will stave off hunger spikes and keep your blood sugar steady. It may not always be possible, but after a while, you will start to notice the difference in how long you feel satisfied.

- **Set a goal of snacking on foods that will make you feel better physically, thus emotionally**. The two go hand in hand. Doing so will lessen the chance of your blood sugar going up and down like a roller coaster. Understand that when you eat foods with simple carbohydrates such as potato chips or a sugar cookie, that is going to get hormones cranking, and lead to more hunger.

- **It's not about giving up your favorites, it's about learning how to live with them.** If you want dessert, an alcoholic beverage, butter on your bread or cream in your coffee, learn how to make a few swaps and strategies. For example, if you are going to be celebrating an occasion, you know there will be dessert. Whether it be before, during, or after, incorporate some foods and behaviors that may help reduce the cravings. Let's say cake is part of the plan. So is a glass of wine. You have found that cake tends to make you hungry for more, and wine reduces your inhibitions. Try having some cheese and crackers, nuts, or half a sandwich with that cake. It's also OK to ask for a smaller portion. Sometimes it can take while to feel the effect of sugar, alcohol and caffeine. After having the dessert and glass of wine, switch off to a glass of water.

Enjoy the celebration and enjoy the energy you have gained from being able to develop new habits and coping mechanisms. If you eat a little more on one day, balance your caloric intake or energy expenditure over the next few days.

- **Commit to yourself to not skip meals.** Skipping meals can send you on a roller coaster of blood sugar highs and lows which tend to cause overeating. Developing a meal pattern of three meals and two or three snack per day will likely keep your hunger levels lower.
- **Breakfast has been shown to help in weight management and help us start our day with more energy.** Often the morning meal is skipped the next day to cut back on calories. Many people skip the morning meal after eating a lot of food the previous day. By midday, they are starved and consequently will be likely to eat more. It will do you good to have something to eat in the morning. You can also make some swaps to cut back on some calories if you have been eating more than usual. Have a fruit salad versus French fries; drink water versus a sweetened beverage; ask for a lowfat sauce on the side in dishes; walk a little longer over the next few days. A few small changes are all it takes. Just a few easy steps and you have achieved success.
- **Studies have shown that learning new activities stimulates the brain.** We live in a time where it is easier to explore new activities. Learning a new language, taking up dancing, or whatever interest you may have can stimulate your brain. You are worth it and you can do it!
- **Check out technology.** There are all types of online applications and mobile devices to help you learn caloric contents of foods, how many calories you need, how much energy you have burned throughout the day, etc.

One online application is *www.meallogger.com*. A few websites include *www.calorieking.com* and *sparkpeople.com* or Google your topic of interest.

- **Think BIG picture**. Things are not going to change overnight or even in a week. Life happens, plans are subject to change. We all overeat at times. It's just a matter of working it off gradually rather than starving oneself for days, which can lead to the cycle of overeating.

Tips for Cravings

We all have cravings. That's part of being human. It's OK to give in to them, and in my opinion, it is important that you do enjoy them on occasion. Food does make us feel good. If crunch and satiety are what you crave, try some pretzels, baked chips, air popped popcorn, or cereal instead of chips. Or, purchase a single serving size of the chips. Some fresh veggies can satisfy the crunch and sweet factor. Carrots, jicama, bell peppers have the crunch and the sweet. Have them with hummus or a dip made with cottage cheese, and add a few herbs or spices such as chives, oregano, rosemary or turmeric. Eating something crunchy can be a great stress reliever!

If it's something sweet you crave, try some fruit with melted dark chocolate and chopped nuts, or some nut butter with fruit such as an apple or banana. Cereal/oatmeal and milk can be a great and satisfying snack. Top it with some cinnamon for the sweet and some nuts for the crunch, fiber, protein and fat. You can even add a little dried fruit. If it's a cookie you crave, accompany it with a glass of ice cold milk, or a cup of sugar-free/plain yogurt.

P.S., if you are making your own cookies, substitute some ground oatmeal for flour to add a little fiber (start by using 1/4 to 1/3 oatmeal to 3/4 to 2/3 flour). Add some nuts as well. Also, try reducing the amount of sugar you use in baked goods or recipes. I have had success in using 1/3 to 1/2 less the amount of sugar in many of my baked goods recipes. You will need to experiment to find out what works for you. If recipe alterations don't work, consider eating smaller portions, such as rounded teaspoons vs. tablespoons when making cookies.

Substitute spices like cinnamon, powdered ginger, cloves, and use extracts like rum, peppermint and the like to reduce the sugar content and add some flavor. Chefs and cooks may gasp at this, but it is worth trying for yourself.

Try a glass of homemade chocolate milk or hot chocolate made with cocoa powder (not instant hot chocolate loaded with added sugar) and a small amount of added sugar/sweetener (not chocolate syrup). You may find that is all the sweetness you need. Many mixes have a lot of added sugar, which adds empty calories. Cocoa powder has antioxidants which contribute to heart health, and has also been shown to create a calming effect.

Recipe
Recipe Acronyms: PRO = protein, CHO = carbohydrate, FAT = fat, Chol = cholesterol

Here's an easy recipe you can make at home or just about anywhere there's hot water. You can touch it up with extracts like peppermint or almond (about 1/4 tsp. per serving), or mix in some ground cinnamon or chili powder.

Easy Cocoa

2 Tbsp. nonfat milk powder

1 tsp. unsweetened cocoa powder

1 tsp. Stevia

In large mug or cup, mix together the milk powder and cocoa.

Add a small amount of water and stir to form a thick consistency and smooth out any lumps.

Add additional water to fill cup to desired serving size.

Heat in microwave for about 1-1/2 minutes.

If desired, make with boiling water versus microwaving.
Makes 1 serving.

Calories per serving: 50 calories 4 gm PRO, 6 gm CHO,
1 gm FAT, 0 mg Chol, 2 gm sugar (from lactose in milk),
25 mg sodium, 183 mg potassium

As silly as it sounds, and as I mentioned before, check out what a three to four ounce piece of cake looks like. I recommend the same strategy for cheese, chips, and whatever it is you crave. Learn what the (proper!) serving size looks like. Weigh it on a food scale, or measure it out in a cup, half, cup, tablespoon, etc. Do this on a regular basis. Keep the visual in your memory. In this way you will become better acquainted with portion sizes. Also, check out *www.measureupbowl.com* for products that can help you learn portion sizes.

If you are reaching for something to do, forget the food, and try getting involved in something else. If you need to chew, try popping a piece of sugarless gum in your mouth and steer away from the kitchen.

When you have the time to strategize, write down a few things you might want to try. Or, write down in your journal what worked in a particular situation. Refer back to that for future reference.

Chapter 6

Back to the Basics

Body Weight

We keep hearing about cutting back on calories, portion sizes and the like, but many of us don't even know how many calories we need per day. Our caloric needs are based on our body weight and activity level. A common form of assessing body weight is the Body Mass Index (see Appendix A). You can also download the BMI calculator to your iPhone at *www.apps.usa.gov/bmi-app*.

BMI Categories

- Underweight = <18.5
- Normal weight = 18.5-24.9
- Overweight = 25-29.9
- Obesity = BMI of 30 or greater[1]

The weight charts give you a starting point. Many in the healthcare community feel that BMI alone is not the only indicator when it comes to risk factors for certain health conditions. There are a few other indicators many healthcare practitioners also refer to. The first is body shape: an apple shape presents for a greater risk of cancer, cardiovascular disease, Type 2 diabetes, metabolic syndrome, and obesity, as more body fat is stored above the hips. A pear shape has more body fat distribution at or below the hips, which are farther away from organs such as the heart, liver and pancreas The second indicator is waist circumference: males with a waist circumference over 40 inches and females with a waist circumference over 35 inches have greater risk for the above mentioned conditions.[2-5]

> **Nutrition Note:** As little as a five to ten percent weight loss can decrease your cardiovascular risk factors. Decreasing your caloric intake by as little as 50 calories per day can result in a loss of five pounds per year; 100 fewer calories per day can result in ten pounds. Or, if you want to look at it another way, increasing your energy expenditure by that amount can produce the same result!

As we age, our body composition does change. Muscle mass is reduced. It is a natural process, and can start as early as the thirties. The key is keeping our muscles active by aerobic exercise and weight lifting to maintain existing muscle mass. The more muscle mass we have, the higher our metabolic rate. Dieting alone will not boost muscle mass. When planning any type of weight loss, exercise is essential in maintaining muscle mass.

Daily Caloric Requirements

One of the things we boomers are starting to experience is the change in our metabolism. We are slowing down. Therefore, we've got to accommodate those changes. We can't eat like we used to without adjusting the portions and increasing our activity level. On average, our caloric needs decline about two percent per decade after we reach adulthood.[6] That whole deal does not seem fair to me. We go through the whole ritual of growing up and then once we're there, we start to slow down?!

Part of the reason, is as mentioned earlier, we start to lose muscle mass. Hormonal changes can also slow our metabolism down a bit as well.[7] Increasing your metabolism doesn't have to be a huge undertaking. We can adjust to these changes in one of two ways—eat less or move more. The great thing is you can mix and match what works for you and give your lifestyle a little variety. We can also incorporate both into our lifestyle. The choice is yours.

The easiest way to calculate your daily caloric needs based on your age, gender and activity level is to go *www.healthfinder.gov/prevention/ViewTopic.aspx?topicID=25&areaID=1*. For those utilizing mobile phone apps, check out *www.meallogger.com*.

The next step is to review the information with a registered dietitian to fine-tune your specific goals. Another easy method to calculate your basal metabolic rate (BMR) is to estimate 10 calories per pound for women and 11 calories per pound for men.[8] BMR does not include activities such as exercise. In the Exercise chapter (Chapter 7) are tips to estimate adding additional calories for activity.

Calorie Counting Note: It takes 3500 calories to lose or gain one pound of body fat. So for those of you out there on numerous "diet regimens," take heed. It is normal for your daily weight to fluctuate.

For example, two cups of water weighs one pound. Some foods, including alcohol, along with hormonal fluctuations can cause initial fluid retention. Foods with high sodium content can cause fluid retention. Even exercise can. Look at the big picture. If you choose to weigh yourself every day, understand body weight is likely to fluctuate within a few pounds.

Now let's take a look at the three main components making up calories in food: Protein, carbohydrates, and fat. There is also a fourth caloric contributor to some of our diets—alcohol. We will also review fiber—what it is, what it does and how it is a positive contributor to our daily diets.

Protein

Comprised of amino acids, protein is a building block.[9] It contains nitrogen, which makes it unique in that it builds and repairs tissue, assists in the production of hormones and digestive enzymes and helps build our immune system. It is a necessary source of energy, containing four calories per gram.[10] Since we lose muscle mass as we age, consuming adequate protein is essential.[11,12] The suggested amount of protein to consume is 15 to 35 percent of your total daily caloric needs.[13]

Looking at it from a body weight perspective, 0.36 grams/lb of body weight for an adult is about right.[14] *To make it easy, a healthy individual's minimum daily protein requirement is about a third of your numerical body weight in grams.* For example, if you weigh 150 pounds, your daily protein needs for an average individual is around 50 to 54 grams.

150 pounds x 0.36 grams/lb of body weight =
54 grams of protein per day.

Athletes and body builders need a little more due to the increased stress on the body, about 0.45 to 0.67gm/lb of body weight.[15] For those individuals, figure a little less than half your body weight in grams of protein. For example, if you weigh 250 pounds,

250 x 0.55 (which is the midpoint between 0.45 to 0.67) =
138 grams of protein per day.

The elderly need a bit more as well, due to the liver's reduced efficiency in producing protein from available amino acids.[16] Pregnant women's protein intake ranges from 60 to 100 grams/day depending on their body weight and specific needs.[17] Discussing your specific needs with your healthcare practitioner or registered dietitian is suggested. Keep in mind, the body only utilizes what it needs. Excess protein is not stored as muscle; it is stored as fat.[18]

A number of studies have suggested that consuming a diet adequate in protein provides for better satiety, body composition (a higher ratio of muscle/fat), and improved blood sugar control.[19-21] And since we lose muscle mass with each decade, the potential for decreased muscle strength is a possibility. Therefore it is important to eat well. This will ensure consuming adequate protein to maintain adequate muscle mass.[22-29]

Types of Protein

Proteins are essentially combinations of different amino acids. There are essential and nonessential amino acids. While the body does produce some nonessential amino acids, it does not produce all the essential amino acids which are needed.[30] Therefore it is necessary to consume additional sources of protein. There are two types of protein: **complete** and **incomplete**:

1. **Complete proteins**—They contain all the essential amino acids necessary for the body's needs. Examples include:
   - ❖ Animal products, such as eggs, chicken, beef, poultry, lamb, seafood and dairy.
   - ❖ Vegetarian products such as tofu, soybeans, tempeh, soy milk and textured vegetable protein (TVP).[31]
2. **Incomplete proteins**—They contain some but not all of the essential amino acids. Examples include:

❖ Plant sources such as beans (kidney, black, pinto, garbanzo, white), legumes, grains, vegetables and nuts.[32]

Vegetarians need to be sure they consume a variety of foods throughout the day to provide all of the essential amino acids. It is not necessary to consume *complementary* proteins at each meal as was once thought. Complementary proteins are formed when two or more foods combine to provide essential amino acids.[33] A few examples of these *complete* combinations include rice with beans (kidney, black, garbanzo, white, red, pinto, etc.), peanut butter on whole wheat bread and macaroni and cheese.

As measurements of protein are going to vary, please refer to the American Diabetes Association website and food advisor at *www.diabetes.org/food-and-fitness/food/my-food-advisor/* and click on the words *My Food Advisor* (this website can also help with analyzing approximate nutrition content of mixed dishes), or go to *www.nhlbi.nih.gov/health/public/heart/obesity/lose_wt/fd_exch.htm*.

To assist in menu planning go to the interactive menu planner at *www.hp2010.nhlbihin.net/menuplanner/menu.cgi*.

Carbohydrates

A carbohydrate is a unit of energy. Each molecule is made up of carbon, hydrogen, and oxygen (thus *carbo* from carbon, and *hydrate* from hydrogen and oxygen).[34] Foods containing carbohydrates contain fiber, sugars and starches, which supply energy in the form of glucose. Glucose is the immediate form of energy utilized by the body. It is also the preferred energy source for the brain and nervous system.[35] Carbohydrate not used immediately for energy is stored in the liver and muscle as glycogen.[36] Excess is stored as fat. Carbohydrates contain four calories per gram.[37] There are two types: **simple and complex.**[38]

Types of Carbohydrates

1. **Simple carbohydrates**—They are those that break down quickly (hence the name simple). Their composition has fewer chemical bonds. Because simple carbohydrates are a smaller molecule, the body digests and absorbs them faster.[39] Consequently, they can make blood sugar rise and fall quickly. When blood sugar rises, the pancreas turns on and secretes insulin to help metabolize glucose. When insulin levels are raised, this causes our body to crave more food to help utilize the insulin. It starts a hunger and response cycle. This cycle can lead to overeating, because our bodies are truly "craving for more."

   Another name for carbohydrates is *saccharides*. There are three types: mono, di, and polysaccharides. Mono and disaccharides are simple carbohydrates. Monosaccharides include glucose, fructose, and galactose. When monosaccharides pair up with each other, they form disaccharides. Disaccharides can take a little longer than monosaccharides to break down, but they are still metabolized quickly. A few examples of disaccharides include sucrose, lactose, and maltose. Sucrose is a naturally occurring sugar in some fruits and some vegetables. It is also commonly known as "table sugar." Lactose is a naturally occurring sugar in milk. Fructose is the naturally occurring sugar found in fruits and honey.[40] Sources of simple carbohydrates include:

   ❖ white bread
   ❖ white sugar
   ❖ white rice
   ❖ processed foods with the fiber and starch stripped

❖ sweetened beverages
❖ fruit juices with added sugar*
❖ sweets such as candy, jello, popsicles, desserts, etc.

Sugars are added to foods under different names. Listed below are additional sources of added sugar.[41]

• Brown sugar	• Invert sugar
• Corn sweetener	• Lactose
• Corn syrup	• Maltose
• Dextrose	• Malt Syrup
• Fructose	• Molasses
• Fruit juice concentrates	• Raw sugar
• Glucose	• Sucrose
• High-fructose corn syrup	• Sugar
• Honey	• Syrup

http://www.cnpp.usda.gov/Publications/DietaryGuidelines/2010/PolicyDoc/PolicyDoc.pdf p. 75.

2. **Complex carbohydrates**—They are just like the name implies. They are made of more complex chains of carbon, hydrogen, and oxygen. Complex carbohydrates are also known as polysaccharides, because they are basically a chain of three or more simple sugars and are therefore a larger molecule. They include starches and fiber and take longer to digest.[42]

Consuming complex carbohydrates are beneficial in so many ways. They have more fiber, which is healthy for the heart and digestive system; maintain blood sugar for a longer period of time; and provide quick and sustained energy. Additionally, complex carbohydrates contain the essential vitamins, minerals and antioxidants we need every day. They also are a satisfying food source.

Think of how many comfort foods contain carbohydrates. If we weren't supposed to eat them, they wouldn't exist. It's really about being more selective in the type of carbohydrate versus the quantity. Sources of complex carbohydrates include:

❖ Fruits*
❖ Vegetables
❖ Whole Grains (whole wheat, rye, barley, oats, flaxseed, quinoa, brown rice, wild rice).[43]
❖ Some vegetarian sources of protein also contain carbohydrates as well. Examples include soy products, beans, nuts and nut butters.

How can fruit juice be a simple carbohydrate and fruits be complex? Many fruit juices are processed and have the skins and fiber removed. Many juices also have added sugar. It can also take two to three times the amount of fruit to make a six to eight ounce glass of juice. Fresh fruits are still intact and have fiber. Keep in mind to check the label on canned fruits, as some may have added syrup/sugars. Look for canned fruits packed in water or in their own juice. If you do buy fruits canned with added syrup or sugars, you can drain or rinse the syrup from the fruit.

3. **The Low Carb Lowdown**—We boomers have seen the low carbohydrate regimens come and go a number of times. There are points to be made regarding this type of regimen. Initially in the first few days when carbohydrate consumption is reduced or eliminated, the body will utilize glucose and glycogen for energy. After depleting glucose and glycogen reserves, if carbohydrates are not consumed, the body will utilize its next easiest energy reserve—muscle.

When muscle is used for energy, electrolyte imbalance can occur. The heart is a muscle, and needs electrolytes. When the electrolyte balance is thrown off enough, it can be fatal. Muscle contains more water and weighs more than fat. When we pull from those reserves we tend to see a quicker drop in our body weight on the scale. This is why. While calories are primarily consumed in the form of protein and fat from meats, cheeses, eggs, butter, oils, etc., they take longer to digest and don't provide that instant energy and glucose as does a carbohydrate. Short term, this type of regimen may assist in lowering blood sugar and body weight. Long term however, these types of regimens do not provide adequate nutrition for the body.

Many people who follow a very low carbohydrate regimen (which may be 20 to 30 percent of calories) for a period of time also find their energy levels are not the same as when eating carbohydrates. As mentioned earlier, the brain relies primarily on blood glucose for energy. So do red blood cells and the nervous system. Carbohydrates are a necessary part of the diet. They provide quick energy and nutrients. It is important to incorporate carbohydrates into your daily eating regimen.[44] And, consuming an adequate amount, may also help maintain a more positive attitude!

A study performed in Australia revealed that individuals who consumed a diet higher in carbohydrates sustained a more positive attitude versus those on a low carbohydrate regimen. One hundred six overweight/obese individuals whose average age was 50 were studied for a year. Participants were divided into two groups: 55 consumed a low carbohydrate, high fat diet (4 percent carbohydrate, 35 percent protein, and

61 percent fat with 20 percent being saturated); 51 consumed a high carbohydrate, lowfat diet (46 percent carbohydrate, 24 percent protein, 30 percent fat, with 8 percent being saturated fat).

During the study, measurements included cognition, mood, anger-hostility, and depression. In the first two months, both groups lost weight (~ 30 lbs.) and experienced an improved outlook. No real secret there, eh?

The researchers noted that both groups followed a specific regimen which included counseling. However, as time progressed, those who consumed the lowfat diet maintained a better state of mind than those on the low carbohydrate diet who tended to be more negative.[45,46]

A few reasons for such a difference were postulated by the researchers. Following a low carbohydrate diet may be difficult in the long term, especially for those on a Western type diet which includes more carbohydrates. Living with the type of structure a low carbohydrate regimen entails can be difficult to maintain, particularly in social situations. The low carbohydrate diet also had an effect on serotogenic functions in the brain. These functions have been associated with depression and anxiety. Conversely, a high carbohydrate diet can potentially increase serotonin synthesis.

Here's what happens: Serotonin is manufactured in the brain and acts like a neurotransmitter. It is synthesized in the body by the amino acid tryptophan and the enzyme tryptophan hydroxylase, which forms 5-hydroxytryptamine, also known as serotonin. Foods high in protein, such as beef, poultry, dairy, nuts, etc. contain higher levels of tryptophan. After an individual consumes a meal high in these proteins, the tryptophan levels actually drop. The reason is that tryptophan is an amino acid and competes with other amino acids to enter the brain. Consequently, only a small amount of tryptophan actually enters the brain, so serotonin levels do not increase.[47]

However, when a higher carbohydrate meal is consumed, it causes the body to release insulin. With a rise in insulin more amino acids are absorbed into the body but not the brain. One exception is tryptophan, which remains elevated and therefore a higher proportion can enter the brain increasing serotonin levels. Another key to help open the door to serotonin synthesis is an adequate supply of vitamin B6 (found in chicken, fish, pork, liver, kidney, whole grains, legumes, and nuts).[48-50]

In summary, if you want to be a little "happier" while reducing your caloric intake, consuming a higher quantity of complex carbohydrates would likely be the ticket. And, remember the combo effect of protein, carbs, fat and fiber make for a perfect combination. Here are a few examples:

- Whole or half sandwich
- Fruit, veggies or crackers with cheese, cottage cheese, hummus or nut butter
- Bowl of oatmeal or cereal with milk
- Unsweetened yogurt with cereal, nuts, and fresh or dried fruit, topped with cinnamon
- A small salad with greens, fresh chopped herbs, veggies, beans (such as black, garbanzo, kidney) and vinegar with a drizzle of olive or canola oil
- A small taco or quesadilla

- Chocolate milk
- Broth based soup with vegetables and protein

Daily consumption of carbohydrates should be around 45 to 65 percent of your daily caloric intake.[51] For example, if daily caloric needs are 1500 calories:

1500 x 0.50 (50%) = 750 calories from carbohydrates
Taking that a step further,
carbohydrates have four calories per gram.
750 calories divided by 4 = 188 grams of carbohydrate per day.

What are serving sizes for carbohydrates? As measurements of carbohydrate will vary, refer to the American Diabetes Association website and food advisor at *www.diabetes.org/food-and-fitness/food/my-food-advisor/* and click on the words *My Food Advisor* (this website can also help with analyzing approximate nutrition content of mixed dishes), or go to *www.nhlbi.nih.gov/health/public/heart/obesity/lose_wt/fd_exch.htm.*

To assist in menu planning go to the interactive menu planner at *www.hp2010.nhlbihin.net/menuplanner/menu.cgi.*

Glycogen and fat need aerobic exercise to wake them up from storage and be converted to energy. Fat burns in the flame of oxygen, meaning aerobic exercise. There is no other way known and proven at this time to shrink fat cells other than aerobic exercise. Men luck out in the weight loss quest, as they are made up of more muscle, and women have more fat mass. More of this will be reviewed in the Exercise section.[52]

Nutrition Note: Many cereals are fortified with vitamins and minerals, some with 100 percent of our daily recommended intake. If you are taking supplementation, perhaps taking them at another meal may be of benefit. The body can only absorb so much at a time and the remainder is excreted.

Fat

Also known as a lipid, fat is a compound made of glycerol (a small water-soluble carbohydrate) and fatty acid. Along with being subjected to a number of transformations, this poor compound has been beaten up and misunderstood. Fat has a number of functions. These include:

- An energy source, providing nine calories per gram.
- Playing a vital role in our bodily functions.
- Promoting the absorption of fat soluble vitamins (A, D, E, and K).
- Playing a role in cell membrane structure, hormonal function and digestion.
- Protecting our body organs and providing insulation in the form of body fat.[53,54]
- Providing flavor to our foods, along with satiety.
- Longer digestion time, thus lessening those hunger pangs and blood sugar fluctuations.

Types of Fats

There are two types of fats: **Saturated and Unsaturated.**

1. **Saturated Fats**—Saturated fats are solid at room temperature. Sources include: fat from animal products such as the fat on meats, skin on chicken, fat in cheese and

dairy products, butter, stick margarine, lard and tropical oils such as coconut, palm and palm kernel oils.[55,56]

Another way to think of saturated fats is that they are saturated with all the hydrogen they can hold. They are one of the fats that can raise blood cholesterol. Anytime you see the word hydrogenated on a label it is a fat that has been "trans" formed into a more saturated fat, thus **trans fats** are formed. Many trans fats start off as a polyunsaturated fat, but through processing, hydrogen is added, thus adding saturation. On a scientific basis, the molecule is also switched from one form to another (a cis isomer to a trans isomer). This process usually occurs during the manufacturing of foods, such as baked goods or fried foods.

These fats are used to extend the shelf life of foods, or act as emulsifiers to keep foods blended. They have a higher smoke point for frying, which has made them appealing to the restaurant industry. In light of more recent and developing health concerns, trans fats have been eliminated from restaurants, thus food manufacturers have had to respond by removing trans fats from their products.

Saturated fats have been linked with an increase of LDL cholesterol levels (low density lipoproteins [LDLs]). LDLs are what stick to the walls of the arteries, potentially causing atherosclerosis and a decrease of HDL cholesterol (high density lipoproteins [HDLs] which assist in clearing fat out of the body).[57,58]

2. **Unsaturated Fats**—Unsaturated fats are those with at least one unsaturated bond (at least one less hydrogen pair). There are two types—polyunsaturated and monounsaturated.

Researchers at Wake Forest University fed monkeys the same number of calories over a six year period; some with monounsaturated fat and some with trans fats. The result was the monkeys in the trans fat group gained four times more weight and it settled in the abdomen.[59]

Polyunsaturated fats have at least two or more missing hydrogen pairs.[60] These fats can help lower cholesterol, along with those pesky LDL guys. They are liquid at room temperature.

Sources of polyunsaturated fats include nuts, seeds and oils such as soy, safflower, sesame, corn, sunflower.[61,62]

Included in the fat picture are fatty acids, and some are essential. Fatty acids are molecules made up of carbon, hydrogen, and oxygen. The body does produce some. Two essential fatty acids the body does not produce however, are linoleic (an omega-6 fatty acid), and alpha-linolenic (an omega-3 fatty acid). Omega-6 fatty acids are a polyunsaturated fatty acid, and found in vegetable and seed oils.

The tricky thing about these fats is they may not only lower LDL, they may also lower HDL.[63-65]

Omega-3 fatty acids are another polyunsaturated fat that has been of much nutritional interest—they have been shown to play an important role in our health. Areas of promise are discussed throughout this book. One example of the effect of omega-3 fatty acids is in their ability to play a role in lowering cholesterol and triglycerides.

In some individuals, however, omega-3 fatty acids may actually raise LDL levels. The rise is due to the particle size, meaning larger particles of LDL versus smaller particles. The smaller particles are more dense and potentially atherogenic (artery clogging), versus the larger particles which are more buoyant. The more buoyant the particle, chances are the less likely the particles will infiltrate the walls of the arteries, which is a good thing.[66-69]

Sources of omega-3 fatty acids include walnuts, flax, chia seeds, fatty fish (such as salmon, mackerel, albacore tuna, sardines, swordfish, lake trout, Atlantic herring, and halibut), canola and soybean oil.[70-75] Supplements containing fish oil are also a good source.[76-82]

For many, the fishy taste of fish oil supplements can be a turn-off. There is a variety of omega-3 fatty acid sources available, ranging from enteric coated capsules, flavored liquid omega fatty acids, and those with a pudding like texture with flavoring added. Many of these products give no fishy aftertaste. Also check on the label for confirmation regarding screening of mercury content.

The American Heart Association website has an updated listing of recommended daily intake, omega-3 fatty acid (and mercury) content in some popular fish/seafood. Access it by going to *www.americanheart.org* and type in *Fish 101.*[83]

As of yet, the United States does not have a recommended intake for omega-3 fatty acids. The World Health Organization and North Atlantic Treaty Organization, however, have made recommendations for omega-3 fatty acids. They are 0.3 to 0.6 gm/day of EPA + DHA, and 0.8 to 1.1 gm/day of alpha-linolenic acid.[84]

Nutrition Note: Regarding mercury—some fish have been linked to the presence of environmental contaminants such as mercury, dioxins, etc. Mercury is a naturally occurring element. In its insoluble form, it is harmless. In its soluble form (which occurs due to industrialization processes, etc.), methyl mercury is poisonous. It is toxic to humans and mammals. In its soluble form, it is easily absorbed, but not easily eliminated. Neurotoxicity is one of the more common outcomes from mercury poisoning. It can damage the brain in developing organisms. Keep in mind that the larger fish are more likely to have higher levels. These fish include tuna, swordfish, king mackerel, tilefish, and shark. The Food and Drug Administration (FDA) and Environmental Protection Agency (EPA) have established that high risk individuals (women who are pregnant or nursing, and very young children) should limit their intake of mercury containing fish to no more than 12 ounces per week of canned light tuna or 6 ounces per week of albacore tuna. Otherwise, for the rest of us, eating fish a few times per week should pose no harm.[85]

Monounsaturated fats are lacking at least one hydrogen pair (hence the word mono). These fats have the potential to lower cholesterol, and possibly raise HDL (the good guys that clear the bad guy LDLs out of your body). Sources include olives, olive oil, canola oil, avocado, and most nuts with the exception of macadamia nuts fried in coconut oil.[86,87]

Another very important role that fats play is in nerve function. The portion of the brain that regulates neurons has a high level of unsaturated, essential fatty acids. Taking this a step farther, there may be a link between the omega-3 fatty acids eicosapentaenoic (EPA) and docosahexaenoic acid (DHA) and mood disorders. Consuming or supplementing the diet with omega-3 fatty acids may be of benefit in some of these conditions.[88-91] More exciting news about omega-3 fatty acids is that research has shown they may play a role in many conditions: reducing inflammation, antiarryhthmic action (that has to with the rhythm of the heartbeat), contribute to control of coronary heart diseases, hypertension, diabetes, autoimmune disorders, atopic eczema, Alzheimer's, dementia, depression, schizophrenia, and multiple sclerosis.[92-98]

3. **Alternatives and their affect on fat metabolism**—With all of the information and confusion regarding fats, there are some alternate sources that can be of benefit. One is plant sterols. They are not a fat. Plant sterols have a similar molecular make up to cholesterol (hence the name sterol).[99] They are naturally occurring in some foods. It is thought that because these molecules are similar to cholesterol, they possibly reduce the absorption of cholesterol.[100] For some individuals, studies have shown that a diet with sterols can lower LDL cholesterol from 6 to 15 percent.[101,102]

     Sources of sterols include almonds, avocado, corn oil, olive oil, soybeans, sunflower seeds and foods with added sterols, such as orange juice, cereal bars, and vegetable oil spreads (margarines).[103] Look for plant sterols on labels and in ingredient listings.

     The American Dietetic Association recommends that for individuals with elevated cholesterol, consumption of 2 to 3 grams per day of plant sterols along with a heart healthy regimen.[104] Try substituting the vegetable oil spreads for butter on occasion in breads, hot cereals, baked goods, rice, potatoes and vegetables. For more information, go to *www.usda.gov* and type in plant sterols for your search. Also discuss the use of plant sterols with your healthcare practitioner.

Another source of fat that is somewhat new to the United States food industry is an oil called Enova.[105] It consists of soy and canola oil. It also contains diacylglycerols/diglycerides (DAG). Conventional oils are made up of triacylglycerols/triglycerides (TAG). DAG oil is manufactured through a process that takes glycerol and fatty acids from canola and soybean oil. These fatty acids are then linked with glycerol to form a diacylglycerol (DAG). Since DAG's have a different shape, the intestines don't build them into a fat molecule like a TAG. Therefore, less fat is absorbed. There have been some studies that have shown it may help in reducing blood and body fat levels. The product has been studied for over 15 years in Japan and in the United States, and has been shown to be safe. It is not a fat substitute. It still has 120 calories per tablespoon, is about 4 percent saturated, and has no trans fats. It has a smoke point of 420°F, so can be used for frying, baking, etc.[106]

4. **Fats in Circulation and Storage—Triglycerides**
   Triglycerides are a form of fat found in our bodies and in foods. They consist of a base of glycerol and three fatty acids. Much of our body fat is stored in the form of triglycerides. They are also the main type of fat that circulates in the blood. Glycerol assists in the transport of fats. Some individuals tend to have higher levels of triglycerides. This can be due to a high intake of

concentrated sweets or alcohol. For others, it can be hereditary or a sign of something else brewing.[107,108] If your triglyceride level is elevated, work with your healthcare practitioner to learn methods of reducing it.

When the majority of us hear fat, we think cholesterol. **Cholesterol** is actually not a fat. It is a waxy substance that our own bodies produce. It is found only in animal sources it is produced in the liver. It too plays a necessary role in cellular function and hormonal synthesis.[109-111]

There are no calories in cholesterol. Some of us have higher cholesterol levels than others. Elevated cholesterol may also be a result of heredity, dietary intake, being overweight, or lack of physical activity.[112] There are a number of means available to assist in the reduction of cholesterol and blood lipids. While medications are one route, many healthcare practitioners will recommend lifestyle modification as well. This includes reducing fat and cholesterol intake along with incorporating exercise.

Increasing soluble fiber intake is a great help (see Fiber section in this chapter for food sources). Changing the types of fats consumed is recommended. Reducing intake of saturated fat and increasing monounsaturated fat has been shown to help lower cholesterol and LDL levels. Consuming fewer concentrated sweets and more fiber containing complex carbohydrates will help with blood sugar control, which, in turn, will reduce the risk of elevating blood lipids.[113,114] Regular exercise will help lower cholesterol and raise HDL levels. Stress reduction can also be of benefit.[115]

In summary, fat makes the news on a regular basis. Many times it is confusing. First, monounsaturated fats are the heavyweights. They are preferred when it comes to being consumed in higher amounts. Next are the polyunsaturated fats. Saturated fats are the fats we want to reduce in our diets, because they can contribute to coronary heart disease. It should be emphasized here; making choices that are REAL for you are important for the quality of your life. Real butter on a fresh hot piece of bread can't be beat. The same recommendation goes for some baked goods. A little of a good thing in a small quantity can be appreciated. Remember the *quality*, not *quantity*, mindset. Try to start thinking this way. Having what you enjoy but less of it may still keep you in a happy, balanced mode.

Nutrition Note: One thing to think about regarding the "fat picture": it is the fact that fried foods typically have 2 to 4 times the calories of their, what I will call, fresh counterparts (those foods prepared without added fats). Think about a white potato—it has about 20 calories per ounce. A typical baked potato is about 8 ounces, thus 160 calories. In contrast, about 4 ounces of French fries is 300 calories and about 20 grams of fat. White meat chicken (which absorbs more fat than dark meat because it has less fat) has about 35 calories per ounce. A baked or broiled four ounce chicken breast has about 140 calories. In contrast, four ounces of fried chicken/chicken pieces has about 350-400 calories. You can make swaps. Sure, once in while these foods are fine. A steady diet of them does create potential for weight gain, artery clogging—you know the drill. Switching to baked or broiled alternatives can save you calories, help your arteries, and gives you those extra calories to enjoy in some other foods, or just not eat them!

How Much Fat do I Need?

The American Heart Association recommends about 20 to 30 percent of our calories should come from fat.[116] Shoot for seven to ten percent saturated fat, and one to two percent trans fat, with the remainder being poly and mono unsaturated. You need to consume at least 10 percent fat daily in your diet to be sure to ingest a sufficient amount of essential fatty acids.[117,118] If this sounds too confusing, remember, most labeled foods break down the fat content.

Let's do some math to help understand how to calculate fat in your daily food intake. Let's say your daily caloric needs are 1500 calories. You have a goal of eating 30 percent fat. Fat has nine calories per gram, therefore:

$$1500 \times 0.30 \ (30\%) = 450 \text{ calories};$$
$$450 \text{ divided by } 9 = 50 \text{ grams per day.}$$

This is what you want to remember in the overall picture of how much fat to consume.

If you want to get more detailed about it, here goes. Taking that a step further, if it is recommended that we consume 7 to 10 percent saturated fat (of our total daily fat intake), then

$$50 \times 0.07 \ (\text{or } 50 \times 0.10) =$$
$$3.5 \ (\text{or up to } 5.0 \text{ grams per day at 10 percent})$$

Last step of the equation is to calculate the amount of recommended trans fat. Current recommendations are at one percent of total daily fat intake.

$$50 \times 0.01 = 0.5 \text{ grams per day}$$

What is a serving of fat? As measurements of fat will vary, refer to the American Diabetes Association website and food advisor at *www.diabetes.org/food-and-fitness/food/my-food-advisor/* and click on the words *My Food Advisor*. (This website can also help with analyzing approximate nutrition content of mixed dishes), or go to *www.nhlbi.nih.gov/health/public/heart/obesity/lose_wt/fd_exch.htm*. And to assist in menu planning go to the interactive menu planner at *www.hp2010.nhlbihin.net/menuplanner/menu.cgi*.

Remember, we need fat! Cars need oil to work (at least for now) and so do we.

Alcohol

Alcohol consumption makes the news on a regular basis in regards to our health. There is evidence that moderate alcohol consumption may benefit the heart. Alcohol has relaxing properties, so this could be one reason why (stress reduction, thus potentially reducing blood pressure). Evidence also suggests that for some, modest alcohol consumption may increase HDL and reduce LDL from forming.[119]

Many studies have shown the benefit of drinking red wine, in particular, because of the compound resveratrol. Resveratrol is a polyphenolic compound and is found in peanuts, some berries and the skin and seeds of grapes. The compound has been shown to have anti-inflammatory properties, which may inhibit some cancers and be of cardiovascular benefit.[120-123] More extensive studies need to be performed to understand the long term effect and health implications.

Moderate consumption is considered one ounce of alcohol per day for women; one to two ounces per day for men. A measured ounce of alcohol is 1ounce hard liquor such as vodka, scotch, rum, tequila; 4 ounces of wine; 12 ounces of beer.[124] When consumed in large quantities (and even modest quantities for some individuals), alcohol can be damaging to the liver, elevate triglycerides and increase the risk for breast cancer.[125,126] Alcohol consumption has also been linked with cancer of the rectum, throat, mouth and esophagus.[127]

If you choose to partake a wee bit, e.g., during cocktail hour, it is suggested to also consume food with alcohol to slow its absorption. The key to consuming alcohol is moderation and responsibility. Each of us is different, and the effects of alcohol will vary. It is important that you understand your own limits. Information regarding the pros and cons of alcohol consumption is readily available. If you have any doubts or concerns, discuss this with your healthcare practitioner.

Alcohol has seven calories per gram.[128] When calculating the caloric content of an adult average, you can go to: American Diabetes Association website and food advisor at *www.diabetes.org/food-and-fitness/food/my-food-advisor/* and click on the words *My Food Advisor.*

A mixed drink with added juices, sweetened carbonated beverages, drink mixes and the like will have an additional 10 to 20 calories per ounce, depending on what is added. For example, a margarita with 2 ounces of tequila (120 calories), plus 6 ounces of tequila drink (120 calories) is about 240 calories. A 2 ounce martini has 2 ounces of vodka/gin/rum (120 calories) and, depending on the vermouth, maybe 1/2 ounce (30 calories), totaling 150 calories.

Fiber

While fiber is not a direct source of calories, it is present in the foods we eat. Fiber is the indigestible component of a food. It is found primarily in plant products.[129] During the processing of foods, fiber can be stripped. A few examples of foods where some fiber has been stripped include white rice, white flour, fruits and vegetables with their skin and pulp removed. Many people have digestive problems, and it could simply be due to lack of enough fiber. The same is true for energy levels. Many people feel sluggish, and once they increase their fiber intake, they rid their bodies of waste and voila, they have more energy. We can all probably use a little more fiber. Our bodies benefit from fiber in a number of ways. First, most of it is indigestible, so you won't get as many calories from it. Second, the two types of fiber—soluble and insoluble—contribute to our overall health.

Soluble Fiber

Soluble fiber acts like a sponge by absorbing the excess fats and cholesterol in our bodies. It is water soluble and when digested, results in a gel-like substance, and is fermented by colonic bacteria. We have healthy (and unhealthy) bacteria in our digestive tract. The healthy bacteria are called probiotics (see more in the Probiotics section, Chapter 3). A diet high in fiber can help keep our healthy bacteria in balance, thus maintaining our digestive health. Soluble fiber has been found to be of benefit in lowering cholesterol and reduce the risk of heart disease. Sources include apples, barley, beans (such as kidney, pinto, black, etc.), berries, broccoli, Brussels sprouts, carrots, citrus, figs, oats, pears, peas, prunes and psyllium.[130,131]

Insoluble Fiber

Insoluble fiber is the fiber that provides bulk and helps aid digestion. It promotes regularity in bowel movements. It is found in whole wheat, wheat products, cereals, fruits, and vegetables. Since it too is indigestible, it can help keep our blood glucose levels steady for a longer period of time and make us feel fuller longer.[132,133]

Fiber can also benefit those who suffer from Diverticulosis. Diverticulosis is a condition which small pockets, called diverticula, are formed in the lining of the intestines. These pockets can occur as a result of increased pressure on weakened areas of the walls of the intestines. Diverticulosis can occur in individuals consuming a diet low in fiber. The condition is thought to occur as a result of increased pressure in the intestines to move and remove small, hard stool.

Since fiber helps keep things moving and basically does a "house cleaning" of the digestive tract, there's a better chance that increasing fiber intake will help you avert such conditions.[134-136] Maintaining a consistent regimen, consuming adequate fluids along with exercise, rest, and regular bowel movements can help to keep the digestive system healthy. Fiber can also help in weight control.[137,138] When people consume foods higher in fiber, they will feel fuller faster, thus eating less. Also, since some of the food is indigestible, it can result in a lower caloric intake.

According to the American Dietetic Association, the recommended adult daily intake for fiber is 25 grams for women and 38 grams for men.[139] Most Americans *may* eat half that amount on a regular basis.[140] I can tell you from experience in counseling many individuals, that when they start eating more fibrous foods, they have a greater boost in energy, feel and look healthier. When considering increasing fiber intake, take it slow. It takes the body a while to adapt to an increased fiber intake. An increase in wheat and bran will need to be supplemented with additional water to help it move through your system. If not, it can backfire and cause constipation. To increase your fiber intake, here are a few suggestions:

- Grind up some flaxseed and add it to cereals, casseroles, baked goods, meatloaf/meat balls, salads, beverages (like smoothies). Mix it in some spreads and dips. Flaxseed has omega-3 fatty acids, so you can get a double whammy. Try doing the same with bran or wheat germ.
- Substitute some ground oat flour for white flour in recipes.

- Increase fruit and vegetable consumption. The edible skin on produce not only has fiber, it also contains more antioxidants. Fruits and vegetables also have more water, and the combination of the fiber and water in fruits and veggies will make you feel fuller.
- Mix a high fiber cereal with your regular cereal. Add some nuts or dried fruit.
- When eating a sandwich have one slice of white bread, and one of either whole wheat, multigrain, rye, or pumpernickel.
- Snacks like popcorn, oatmeal, whole grain cereals, nuts and dried fruit all contain fiber.

Putting it All Together

You now know your daily caloric, protein, carbohydrate, fat, and fiber needs. Designing a meal plan based on your lifestyle is up to you. There are many resources, such as cookbooks, nutrition books, websites, and classes you can participate in to further your learning. A suggestion you will encounter throughout this book is to eat small frequent meals and to incorporate a mix of protein, carbohydrates, fat and fiber into them. While increasing fruit and vegetable intake is recommended (five plus servings per day), it may be challenging for some to achieve. Make that one goal. Incorporate whole grains into your daily eating pattern. Make the change gradually. Eating more produce, whole grains and fiber will increase your chances of living a healthier life. Cutting back on saturated fats, sugar and sodium will also lend a hand in reducing your risk of developing or complicating conditions such as cancer, cardiovascular disease, diabetes, and metabolic syndrome. Don't let yourself get confused with calculating percentages and grams. Those will all come in time. As you continue reading through *Boomer Be Well!* things will come together to assist you in being more informed and taking charge of your health.

Weight Loss Tip: One thing you may want to consider in the weight loss plan is to estimate how many calories you would need to consume at your goal weight. Discuss this with a registered dietitian or your healthcare practitioner before implementing.

Portion Sizes

Portion sizes are actually very easy to learn. You also know approximate measures for a serving. To effectively learn portion sizes, you will need measuring cups, spoons and a food scale. Once you measure them out and actually see what they look like on a plate or in a bowl, this can help you when you are dining out as well as traveling.

You can also use objects to associate portion sizes. For example, a cooked three ounce portion of meat may look like a deck of cards, a hockey puck, or the size of the palm of your hand; two tablespoons of nut butter is the same size as a golf ball; a cup of rice, pasta or potatoes looks like the size of a baseball. A handful of nuts are about 1/4 cup, which is an ounce. Measure a 1/4 cup of nuts and pour them into your hand; see how much it looks like. Measure out an ounce of cereal and a 1/2 cup or full cup of milk into the cereal bowl. Look at how much is in your bowl. Practice using measuring cups and spoons as serving utensils once in a while to keep a gauge on portions. It is easy for portion sizes to grow larger without keeping an eye on them!

Calculating Combination Foods

Mixed foods are things like casseroles, combination foods, soup, fried rice, etc. Typically, a portion size is one cup. There are a lot of books and websites out there on calories that list just about everything. If you are interested in any of them, they may be great to have as a reference. Most fast food restaurants have calorie charts or brochures with their products listed. Some have websites that can assist you in planning lower calorie meals.

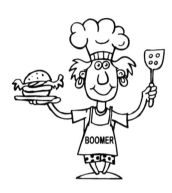

An easy way to learn and understand the caloric content of meals is to break them into ingredients just like a recipe. If you are making the meal, you can easily do this. If it is a packaged product, you can also do it. Utilize the information on the web links to help you categorize foods, such as low, medium, and high fat meats, a tortilla, a cocktail, etc. Here are a few examples using the American Diabetes Association website:

Mexican Combination Meal

2 soft corn tortillas = 120 calories, 2 starch

2/3 c. rice = 150 calories, 2 starch

1/2 c. beans = 100 calories, 1 starch, 1 lean meat

3/4 cup ground/shredded beef/pork/chicken = 210 calories, 3 medium fat meat

1/4 cup grated cheese = 100 calories, 1 high fat meat

2 Tbsp. sour cream = 65 calories, 1 fat

2 Tbsp. guacamole/avocado = 50 calories, 1 fat

Total = 795 calories

If you think the meat was cooked in oil (chances are yes), add another fat or two which will add 50 to 100 calories.

Three Ounce Glazed Doughnut—
A Calorie Calculation

Let's break it down. For example, if a doughnut weighs three ounces (28 gm in an ounce x 3 = 84 gm), figure three pieces/ounces of bread/starch (70 x 3 = 210). It will have added fat as it's fried, about 2 tsp (which will be around 10 gm fat, 90 calories), and also some sugar in the glaze (10 gm, about 40 calories). Our three ounce doughnut comes to:

210 + 90 + 40 = 340 calories

Macaroni and Cheese

1 cup cooked macaroni = 200 calories, 2 starch

Cheese sauce mixture of cheese, milk, flour, butter broken down per serving:

1/4 cup grated cheddar cheese = 100 calories, 1 high fat meat

1 Tbsp. butter = 100 calories, 3 fat

1 Tbsp. flour = 25 calories, 1/3 starch

4 Tbsp. milk (whole) = 35 calories, 1/4 milk

Total = 460 calories per cup/serving

Asian combination meal

1 chicken eggroll =170 calories, 1 starch, 1 lean meat, 1 fat

1 cup Sweet and Sour (pork/chicken) = 450 calories, 2 starch, 2-1/2 other carbohydrate, 1 non-starchy vegetable, 1 lean meat

1 cup fried rice = 300 calories, 2 starch, 2 medium fat meat

1 fortune cookie = 35 calories, 1/2 starch

Total = 955 calories

Look at this as a game, not a chore. It takes a little time and practice to learn. You can go to the websites listed for protein, carbohydrate, fat and alcohol for more help.

Chapter 7

Exercise

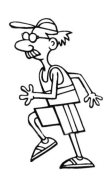

Benefits

Exercise has been shown to promote a wealth of health. A few of these nuggets include:

- Heart health
- Increasing HDL cholesterol levels
- Weight maintenance
- A feeling of well being
- Sharpening our minds
- Keeping our muscles and bones strong
- Lowering blood pressure
- Possible longevity of life
- Relieve stress

Numerous studies support these benefits.[1-4] It is a necessary component in a healthy lifestyle. Thus, if we do want to take care of our bodies, think about how we can incorporate exercise/movement into our lives. Before beginning any type of exercise regimen consult your healthcare practitioner.

As stated earlier, 3500 calories will add or lose one pound of body fat. Decreasing caloric intake either by eating less and/or increasing physical activity will help lose weight. No surprise there.

The recommended rate of healthy weight loss is approximately one half to two pounds per week. The way to keep it off is to maintain or increase physical activity. A lot of people don't fit that piece of the puzzle in that part of their life. We've adapted to what I call technology induced lifestyles. Technology takes care of things we used to do with an expenditure of physical energy. If you think about it, when we boomers were growing up, we had a lot more physical activity. Many of us had fun doing it. We also had time to get other things done. Maybe we can think about meeting halfway with the past and present, get off our fannies and move it. If you can't take time out to take care of yourself, something is definitely off in the balance of your universe. A little surge of endorphins (through exercise) might just bring you back in balance and restore some of that youthful exuberance.

There are three types of exercise: aerobic, weight lifting, and recreational. Aerobic exercise is what gets our blood and heart muscle pumping. Examples of this include brisk walking, cycling, swimming, rollerblading, snowshoeing, jogging, running, and the like. Anything that can increase and sustain our heart rate for 20 to 30 minutes (or more) is considered aerobic exercise. Working up to 30 minutes of physical activity most days of the week is suggested to stay physically fit.[5-8] Some of you may be thinking where and how are you going to get an additional 30 minutes of activity in your day? Break it up if need be. Remember, every day would be ideal, and it does not mean strenuous activity. It's about moving.

Weight lifting is another form of exercise. It can increase muscle mass and strength. By increasing muscle mass, weight lifting can also raise our metabolism. Weight lifting also helps support our bones. It is recommended to lift weights two to three times per week.[9,10] The best way to start is consulting with a trainer/exercise physiologist or physical therapist. These individuals can show the proper mechanics and amount of weight to lift for your specific needs. They can also help you set goals.

Many local recreation centers have fitness programs available to learn weight training techniques. Even though you can research weight lifting on the internet and in books, it is best to have someone show you. It is far too easy to perform a maneuver with poor posture resulting in injury. For information on finding an exercise physiologist in your area, go to *www.asep.org*; for a physical therapist go to *www.apta.org*.

Recreational exercise is what I also call stress management. This includes golf, tennis, racquetball, volleyball, baseball, softball, skiing, soccer, tai chi, gardening and many more. Some of these activities can really get your heart rate going. They also are a fun way to incorporate exercise into your lifestyle.

Strategies for Incorporating Exercise

- Incorporating exercise into your life is going to take some planning and commitment. Many of us have busy lives. Each week may be different. Therefore, take one week at a time. Write down what type of physical activity goals you are going to accomplish and the time of day you are going to fit it in. You can do this either through a journal or a notepad. Keep it readily available. Also have back up plans if you are planning outdoor activities. Mother Nature may not always cooperate.

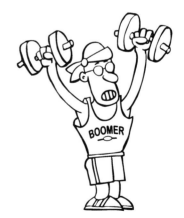

- If you are not someone who wants to join a gym or exercise class, there are many options available. Purchasing or checking exercise CDs out of your local library will provide you with a private exercise session.

- If you do want to join a gym or recreation center, there are classes, equipment and instructors available to assist you.
- Keep an extra pair of sneakers and work-out clothes in your car or office. This way they will always be handy.
- Take advantage of where you are. If you are short on time, but need to run errands, here's a tip: At the grocery or department store, after you have finished shopping and your cart is full, walk up and down every aisle of the store. If some aisles are a temptation for you, walk the perimeter a few times. This may not be the same as a full workout, but you are moving and getting exercise. Do the same in a mall. It is protected from the elements and you can get some mileage in.
- Enlist friends or family to exercise together. This can help prevent boredom along with helping encourage each other to exercise.
- Form a walking group in your neighborhood.
- Walk the dog a little longer each day (or pretend you have one).
- Get up from your desk frequently and walk around. Take the stairs if they are safe.
- During your breaks, get out of the building and get some fresh air if the climate permits.
- Get up and move while watching television. Believe it or not, many people have started and maintained a successful weight loss and fitness program while watching television. Pretend you have a jump rope; do some jumping jacks; walk in place; move your arms.

- Speaking of television, check out the option on cable TV for exercise television. There are a number of exercise classes you can utilize in the privacy of your home and at a convenient time of day.
- When travelling, you can exercise either in the hotel fitness center (if there is one), or work out in your hotel room. Pretend you have a jump rope, do some aerobic exercises, yoga poses, turn on some music, etc.

Chances are there are a few exercises you may really enjoy. Mix your activities up to give you variety. Activity is essential to keeping the body going. Learning to incorporate some type of exercise every day is likely to make you feel better all over.

10,000 Steps

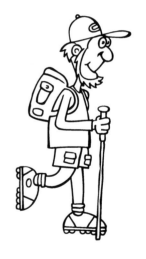

These days, we hear a lot about strapping on a pedometer and setting the goal of walking 10,000 steps in a day. How much is that? 10,000 steps is five miles.[11] If you are just starting an exercise regimen do not expect or attempt to walk 10,000 steps in a day-please! Take it slow. Remember, it takes three to six months to "learn" a new behavior, so give it a chance.

If walking is your prime exercise target, fasten a pedometer on in the morning. Make sure it is fastened to a snugly fitted belt or something like it and worn in a location just above the hip so it can detect the movement of a step. Take it off when you are finished moving around for the day. See what your current level is. You may surprise yourself. Many people find wearing a pedometer is a great motivator.

Energy Expenditure

If you wonder how many calories you burn while exercising there are websites you can refer to based on your specific age, sex, and activity level. Here are a few:

- *www.Healthfinder.gov* has a quick guide to healthy living in the nutrition and fitness section
- *www.bmi-calculator.net/bmr-calculator/harris-benedict-equation*
- *www.mayoclinic.com/health/calorie-calculator/NU00598*
- A few other websites for activity and exercise tips are *www.smallstep.gov* and *www.cdc.gov/healthyweight/physical_activity/index.html*

The accompanying chart provides an estimate of calories expended during exercise. As the chart is based on a body weight of 154 lbs., here's an easy way to calculate your caloric expenditure compared to that of someone weighing 154 lbs:

Divide your weight into 154 lbs. For example if you weigh 200 lbs., divide 200/154. You get a factor of 1.29. Use that factor to multiply the caloric expenditure. Let's use the hiking for 30 minutes activity. Multiply 185 x 1.29 and you get 238. That's approximately how many calories a 200 lb. individual would burn hiking for 30 minutes.

If you weigh 130 lbs., divide 130/154. You get a factor of 0 .84. Let's use the 30 minute hiking activity. Multiply 0.84 x 185 and you get 156. A 130 lb. person would burn approximately 156 calories on a 30 minute hike.

Calories Used per Hour in Common Physical Activities

Moderate Physical Activity	Approximate Calories/30 Minutes for a 154 lb Person[1]	Approximate Calories/Hr for a 154 lb Person[1]
Hiking	185	370
Light gardening/yard work	165	330
Dancing	165	330
Golf (walking and carrying clubs)	165	330
Bicycling (<10 mph)	145	290
Walking (3.5 mph)	140	280
Weight lifting (general light workout)	110	220
Stretching	90	180
Vigorous Physical Activity	Approximate Calories/30 Minutes for a 154 lb Person[1]	Approximate Calories/Hr for a 154 lb Person[1]
Running/jogging (5 mph)	295	590
Bicycling (>10 mph)	295	590
Swimming (slow freestyle laps)	255	510
Aerobics	240	480
Walking (4.5 mph)	230	460
Heavy yard work (chopping wood)	220	440
Weight lifting (vigorous effort)	220	440
Basketball (vigorous)	220	440

[1]Calories burned per hour will be higher for persons who weigh more than 154 lbs (70 kg) and lower for persons who weigh less.

Adapted from *Dietary Guidelines for Americans 2005*, page 16, Table 4.

http://www.health.gov/dietaryguidelines/dga2005/document/html/chapter3.htm#table4.

Chapter 8

Conditions Improved
by Lifestyle

Healthy Lifestyle Recommendations

It really should come as no surprise to us that many health conditions are a result of our lifestyle. Cancer, Cardiovascular Disease, Diabetes, Metabolic Syndrome and Osteoporosis are a few of these conditions. Recommendations from numerous organizations such as the American Cancer Society, American Dietetic Association, American Heart Association, and American Diabetes Association, all have a similar set of suggestions for maintaining a healthy lifestyle. These include:

- Eating more fruits and vegetables
- Increase consumption of whole grains and legumes
- Consume lean meats, poultry, seafood, and lowfat dairy products
- Reduce intake of trans and saturated fats
- Reduce or eliminate intake of concentrated sweets
- Attain and maintain a healthy weight
- Incorporate physical activity/exercise daily (with a goal of 30 minutes per day)
- Consume alcohol in moderation
- If you smoke or use tobacco products, quit

- Choose and prepare foods low in sodium
- Do not rely on dietary supplements to protect against cancer

_____

Adapted from Dietary Guidelines, 2010 National Institute of Health, and American Institute for Cancer Research

In this chapter, we will review a number of conditions linked to lifestyle and discuss strategies to alleviate symptoms and reduce risk factors.

Arthritis

Arthritis is a condition caused by an inflammatory response. The word arthritis means joint inflammation. According to the Center for Disease Control and Prevention, it is the most common cause of disability in the United States.[1]

The term arthritis refers to over 100 rheumatic diseases and conditions that affect joints, the tissues that surround the joint and other connective tissue.[2] There are two common types: Osteoarthritis (OA) and Rheumatoid (RA).[3]

OA is the more common form of arthritis.[4] It occurs due to the cartilage between the joints and bones wearing down, thus causing pain and stiffness. Risk factors include excess body weight (knees are particularly vulnerable), long term stress or injury, muscle weakness, structural malalignment. Women tend to be at greater risk than men for OA. Genetic predisposition, aging, osteoporosis, estrogen deficiency, and elevated C-reactive protein levels are additional factors.[5-11]

Treatment for OA consists of weight management, physical therapy, patient education, and the use of some medications. Some dietary suggestions include adequate vitamin C, vitamin D, calcium and some herbal supplements.[12]

> Did you know a study at Wake Forest University
> revealed that for every pound of weight lost takes four
> pounds of pressure per step off the knees?[13]

RA is a systemic inflammatory disease. It manifests itself in multiple joints of the body but can also affect other organs.[14] RA can begin at any age, and symptoms include prolonged stiffness and fatigue. It is more common in women than men (two to three times higher), and incidence peaks in the 60s. While no definitive causes are known, it is thought that RA may be due to a faulty immune response. Some researchers have looked at genetics and environmental factors (such as hormonal exposures, microbial exposures from bacteria or viruses and tobacco use) as risk factors for RA. Of the environmental factors, use of tobacco has been shown to have a consistent association with the onset of RA.[15]

Some evidence shows a dietary component to RA.[16] Some foods may be regarded as trigger points, and some foods may help alleviate symptoms. Treatment of RA includes medication, surgery in some cases, exercise and self management. There is still much research needed to be definitive for dietary treatment of both OA and RA. As the condition itself is inflammatory, individuals will likely need specific treatment in regards to their individual situation.

Some individuals with arthritis may experience an aggravation of their symptoms with such foods as potatoes, tomatoes, eggplant, peppers and tobacco. These are a group of foods known as nightshades.[17]

Natural anti-inflammatory remedies that have shown promise in pain reduction include cinnamon, ginger, turmeric, cherries, and omega-3 fatty acids. Bromelain is another compound found to be potentially beneficial in maintaining healthy joints and reducing pain.[18-25] One source is pineapple.

Exercise has also been shown to help alleviate some of the pain and symptoms of arthritis, while improving circulation and physical fitness.[26] Some individuals with OA have experienced relief of pain and symptoms with supplements containing chondroitin sulfate, glucosamine sulfate, and others with omega-3 fatty acid supplements. Others have not.[27-29] There are a number of studies to review at *www.webmd.com*.

Check with your healthcare practitioner regarding any use of supplements and physical activity. For more information regarding Arthritis check out *www.cdc.gov/arthritis/basics.htm or www.arthritis.org*.

Recipes

Recipe Acronyms: PRO = Protein; CHO = Carbohydrate;
FAT = Fat; Chol = Cholesterol; Gram = gm

Fish: Baked, Broiled or Grilled

Bake, broil or grill some delicious omega-3 loaded fish such as Salmon, Tuna, Halibut or Mackerel. Season it with a sprinkle of turmeric, black pepper and some citrus juice. Accompany it with some Pineapple Mint Salsa.

Pineapple Mint Salsa

2 cups fresh or 1 can (20-ounces) pineapple chunks in their own juice, drained

2 Tbsp. lemon or lime juice (or you can substitute with rice wine vinegar)

1/4 cup chopped mint

Salt and Pepper to taste

Combine all ingredients. You may want to use a lesser amount of juice/vinegar and taste it before adding more. Cover and refrigerate for at least 30 minutes for flavors to blend. Makes 4 servings.

Per serving: 60 Calories, 1 gm PRO, 15 gm CHO, 0 gm FAT, 0 mg Chol, 1 gm Fiber, 3 mg Sodium, 128 mg Potassium.

Salmon Salad

1 can (7-ounces) boneless, skinless salmon, drained

1 Tbsp. Mayonnaise*

1 stalk celery, preferably organic, chopped

1 tsp. lemon juice

1/4 tsp. ground turmeric

1 tsp. minced fresh ginger or 1/2 tsp. dried, if desired

*You can substitute lower fat mayonnaise or yogurt if preferred, which will reduce calories and fat.

Mix all ingredients in bowl. Refrigerate. Makes 2 servings.

Per serving : 170 Calories, 21 gm PRO, 1 gm CHO, 8 gm FAT, 36 mg Chol, 376 mg Sodium, 266 mg Potassium.

Asthma

A condition where the airways are irritated and/or inflamed, asthma is a response to some type of irritant inhaled, ingested, or absorbed.[30] Sometimes it can be brought on by exercise, a virus, heartburn (gastro esophageal reflux, also known as GERD), sulfites in foods and possibly obesity.[31-33] Additional triggers may include tobacco smoke, weather, pets, medications, cockroaches, dust mites, mold, physical activity, some foods (as mentioned in the food allergy section, Chapter 3) and/or food additives, such as sulfites.[34-37] Treatment for asthma usually involves medication and lifestyle modification.[38]

While more concrete evidence is needed, some studies have shown that some foods, such as those that contain antioxidants in fruits and vegetables, may help alleviate the symptoms of asthma. A few include vitamin C and magnesium.[39-45] Quercetin is one compound that has been found to have potential in alleviating some symptoms and aid in the treatment of asthma. It is found in apples, onions, cherries, celery, and broccoli.[46-47]

Another food source that has emerged as a possible anti-inflammatory agent in asthma is omega-3 fatty acids. Sources of these fatty acids are fatty fish, such as salmon, halibut, mackerel, herring, sardines, and tuna. Plant sources of omega-3 fatty acids include flax and chia seed, walnuts, and canola oil.[48-50] A Mediterranean diet (whole grains, fruits, vegetables, nuts, legumes, fish, and olive oil) may have a protective role in asthma like symptoms and allergic rhinitis in children.[51-52] Consuming foods with omega-3 fatty acids two to three days per week (in four to six ounce portions) may provide some relief. In the meantime, reach for a juicy apple; chew on some crisp celery (perhaps with some cream cheese or nut butter); chop or mince some onions in a salad or dish; indulge in some fresh or dried cherries. At the very least, these foods make a great snack. See "Example of Functional Components Chart" (Chapter 3) for food sources.

For more information regarding Asthma, go to: *www.nhlbi.nih. gov/health/dci/Diseases/Asthma/Asthma_WhatIs.html* or *American Lung Association at www.lungusa.org/.*

A recipe of stewed apples is a simple, yet versatile dish. It makes a great accompaniment to a hot steaming bowl of oatmeal with nuts, adds flavor and texture to a dish of plain yogurt, lends a tangy taste as a side dish with pork, and is also a filling in a pie, or can be served plain.

Sinus Tips: For those with sinus problems, many healthcare practitioners now recommend using a sinus rinse on occasion to help irrigate them. Saline spray may help as well. Additionally, many of us may unknowingly suffer from an allergy to molds, bacteria and fungus. Getting tested can help you find out.

Ask your practitioner about this and other non-prescription remedies.

And did you know that washing your pillow frequently may help alleviate some of the allergens affecting the sinuses? Dust, dander, dust mites, etc. can all inhabit in our pillows. Purchasing washable pillows and washing them on a regular basis (such as once a month) may help alleviate some allergy symptoms.

Recipes

Recipe Acronyms: PRO = Protein; CHO = Carbohydrate; FAT = Fat; Chol = Cholesterol; Gram = gm

Stewed Apples

2 red apples, preferably organic, washed and chopped with skin on

2 Granny Smith apples, preferably organic, washed and chopped with skin on

1 Tbsp. minced fresh ginger, or 2 tsp. powdered ginger

1/2 tsp. cinnamon

Lemon juice to coat apples

Optional: dried cranberries, raisins, dried or fresh pitted cherries

Toss apples with lemon juice.

Place all ingredients in a sauce pan.

Add enough water to cover bottom of pan to prevent scorching. Place lid on saucepan.

Cook over medium heat until apples are soft, about 20 minutes. Serve immediately or refrigerate. Makes 4 servings.

Per serving: 74 Calories, 0.5 gm PRO, 19 gm CHO, 0 gm FAT, 0 mg Chol, 3 gm Fiber, 1 mg Sodium, 159 mg Potassium.

The dish below can make a great accompaniment to meals, breakfast, lunch, dinner or as a snack. Have it for breakfast with cottage cheese and top with walnuts.

Waldorf Salad

2 red apples, preferably organic, washed and chopped

2 Granny Smith apples, preferably organic, washed and chopped

Lemon juice (about 1-2 tsp.)*

1 large celery stalk, preferably organic, washed and chopped

1/4 cup walnuts, chopped

1/4 cup dried or fresh pitted chopped cherries, preferably organic

1/2 cup plain nonfat yogurt strained (drain in a sieve for about 20 to 30 minutes)

1/2 tsp. ground cinnamon

1 tsp. minced fresh ginger (or 1/2 tsp. powdered ginger)

Mix apples with lemon juice (to prevent browning).

Mix all other ingredients together. Refrigerate and let sit for 1 hour or so for flavors to blend. Makes 4 servings.

Per serving: 145 calories, 3 gm PRO, 24 gm CHO, 5 gm FAT, 4 gm Fiber, 1 mg Chol, 33 mg Sodium, 306 mg Potassium.

*If fresh lemons are not available or too expensive, ask your grocer for organic bottled lemon juice. It does not contain added sodium, etc. It will last for months in your refrigerator (and is also cheaper in the long run). You can add it to your drinking water for a refreshing zest, use it as a flavor enhancer, etc.

Cancer

In the normal body process, cells grow and divide on a regular basis. Old or damaged cells are typically replaced with new cells. On occasion, this process can go awry. Compounds known as free radicals can damage cells, resulting in the alteration of DNA (the genetic material of a cell). When this occurs, a process of mutation alters normal cell growth and division. This alteration or mutation of cells can or may result in cancer.[53]

Most cancers are classified by their origin or location. For example, cancer that originates in the colon is called colon cancer. The National Cancer Institute estimates there are over 100 types of cancer.[54] Cancer can spread through the bloodstream or the lymphatic system to other areas of the body. Some cancers may be inherited, while others may result from environmental or lifestyle factors. These factors include:

- Growing older
- Tobacco
- Sunlight
- *Ionizing radiation* (which includes radon gas, radioactive fallout, x-rays)
- Certain chemicals and other substances (asbestos, benzene, vinyl chloride and others)

- Some *viruses* and *bacteria* (such as Human Papilloma Virus (HPV), Hepatitis B and C and others)
- Certain *hormones* (such as estrogen and progestin)
- Alcohol (> 1 drink per day for women and > 2 per day for men)
- Poor diet, lack of physical activity, or being overweight[55]

Reprinted with permission from National Cancer Institute U.S. National Institutes of Health, *www.cancer.gov*.

In 2007, American Institute for Cancer Research (AICR) and its affiliate, the World Cancer Research Fund (WCRF) in the United Kingdom, released the Second Expert Report "*Food, Nutrition, Physical Activity and the Prevention of Cancer: a Global Perspective.*" This international report is the largest of its kind ever published, with more than 7,000 studies analyzed by a 21-member expert panel. According to AICR's Director for Research, Susan Higginbotham, PhD, "The report examines a comprehensive list of 'exposures' related to food, nutrition, physical activity and weight." The report found some of the strongest links to cancer risk are excess body fat and lack of physical activity. Convincing evidence revealed that excess body fat increases the risk of pancreatic, kidney and postmenopausal breast cancer. The theory of excess body fat and its link to certain cancers is that with an increase in fat cells comes an increase in levels of growth factors and hormones. Both can promote the growth of cancer cells.

Additionally, an increase in abdominal fat can lead to an increase in insulin resistance and thus insulin production. The risk of some cancers is increased with high insulin levels. Swedish researchers found that a high sugar intake increases the risk of pancreatic cancer. When high levels of sugar are ingested, insulin and glucose levels rise. And, as previously stated, excess levels of insulin result in "insulin-like growth factor," which can possibly promote cell proliferation and cancer.[56] Chronic inflammation can promote the growth and development of cancer cells; a low level of chronic inflammation can occur with an increase in fat cells. It is also thought that some viral, bacterial, and parasitic infections may cause some long term inflammation. Long term inflammation may suppress the immune system and possibly have an impact on a cell's DNA.

According to the American Cancer Society, about 15 to 20 percent of cancers worldwide are linked to infections.[57] The 2007 report also found regular physical activity may possibly protect against colon, post-menopausal breast and endometrial cancer. In relation to diet, the study found that consuming greater than 18 ounces of red meat per week increased the risk of colorectal cancer. The reasons why are not clear, as the causes may stem from the preparation of red meat at high heat (such as pan-fried or well-done) to compounds created when meats are processed such as in curing or smoking.[58]

A report published in the medical journal *The Lancet*, stated that 35 percent of the seven million deaths from cancer in 2001 were caused by a lifestyle that could have been changed. The study drew attention to modifiable risk factors. These factors include fruit and vegetable intake, smoking, alcohol use, overweight, and obesity.[59]

In regards to foods and their relation to cancer risk reduction, as stated in the Examples of Functional Component Chart (Chapter 3), those food groups with a higher antioxidant level can help boost our immune system and neutralize free radicals. Additionally, foods with insoluble fibers can aid in digestion and elimination. A few examples listed in the chart include consuming foods that help neutralize free radicals and boost defenses.

Cancer can be detected at any stage. Early detection is important. Perform monthly examinations of breast, skin, mouth, and testicles. Have annual physical examinations. The cancer screening process can be based on a number of factors. Some include age, symptoms, family history, lifestyle, and risk of procedure. Cancer treatment is more effective when found in the early stage of the disease. Discuss any changes in your body or health status with your healthcare practitioner and also discuss cancer screening with him or her.[60] The National Cancer Institute recommends:

- **Breast:** A *mammogram* is the best tool doctors have to find breast cancer early. A mammogram is a picture of the breast made with x-rays. The NCI recommends that women in their forties and older have mammograms every one to two years. Women who are at higher-than-average risk of breast cancer should talk with their healthcare practitioner about whether to have mammograms before age 40 and how often to have them. Those at higher risk for breast cancer may also be screened by magnetic resonance imaging (MRI) in addition to a mammogram.[61]
- **Cervix:** The *Pap test* (sometimes called Pap smear) is used to check cells from the cervix. The doctor scrapes a sample of cells from the cervix. A lab checks the cells for cancer or changes that may lead to cancer (including changes caused by human papilloma virus, the most important risk factor for cancer of the cervix). Women should begin having Pap tests three years after they begin having sexual intercourse, or when they reach age 21 (whichever comes first). Most women should have a Pap test at least once every three years.
- **Colon and rectum:** A number of screening tests are used to detect *polyps* (growths), cancer or other problems in the colon and rectum. People aged 50 and older should be screened. People who have a higher-than-average risk of

cancer of the colon or rectum should talk with their doctor about whether to have screening tests before age 50 and how often to have them.

- **Fecal occult blood test:** Sometimes cancer or polyps bleed. This test can detect tiny amounts of blood in the stool.
- **Sigmoidoscopy:** The doctor checks inside the rectum and lower part of the colon with a lighted tube called a sigmoidoscope. The doctor can usually remove polyps through the tube.
- **Colonoscopy:** The doctor examines inside the rectum and entire colon using a long, lighted tube called a colonoscope. The doctor can usually remove polyps through the tube.
- **Double-contrast barium enema:** This procedure involves several x-rays of the colon and rectum. The patient is given an enema with a barium solution, and air is pumped into the rectum. The barium and air improve the x-ray images of the colon and rectum.
- **Digital rectal exam:** A rectal exam is often part of a routine physical exam. The healthcare practitioner inserts a lubricated, gloved finger into the rectum to feel for abnormal areas. A digital rectal exam allows for examination of only the lowest part of the rectum.

Reprinted with permission National Cancer Institute, U.S. National Institutes of Health *www.cancer.gov/cancertopics/wyntk/overview/page5.*

Websites for additional cancer information include:
The National Cancer Institute *www.cancer.gov*
The American Cancer Society *www.cancer.org*
The American Institute for Cancer Research *www.aicr.org*

Recipes

Recipe Acronyms: PRO = Protein; CHO = Carbohydrate;
FAT = Fat; Chol = Cholesterol; Gram = gm

Following are a few recipes loaded with antioxidants and flavor.

Berry Medley Surprise

In addition to enjoying this dish on its own, it also makes a great topping to angel food cake, ice cream, plain yogurt, and as a filling in pies or a fruit tart.

2 cartons (6-ounces each) fresh raspberries, preferably organic

1 pint fresh blueberries, preferably organic

or substitute 5 cups frozen mixed berries, thawed

1.5 ounces dark chocolate (60% cacao) chopped into small bite-size pieces

1/4 cup chopped nuts

1 tsp. minced fresh ginger

1 tsp. cinnamon

Mix nuts, cinnamon and ginger. Set aside.

Divide berries into 6 microwaveable dishes.

Divide chopped chocolate evenly among dishes.

Microwave for about 20 seconds (or until chocolate is soft). Top with nut mixture.

If you like, you can toast the nuts on a cookie sheet for 5 to 10 minutes under a broiler to give them a roasted flavor. Makes 6 servings.

Per serving: 160 Calories, 3 gm PRO, 27 gm CHO, 6 gm FAT, 0 gm Chol, 9 gm Fiber, 2 mg Sodium, 264 mg Potassium.

Mediterranean Vegetable Mix

1 small onion, chopped

2 cloves garlic, chopped

1 Tbsp. olive, canola, or Enova oil

1 Tbsp. fresh minced (or 2 tsp. dried) ginger

1 Tbsp. fresh minced (or 2 tsp. dried) oregano

1 Tbsp. fresh minced (or 2 tsp. dried) basil

3/4 pound fresh broccoli, broken into pieces

1 can (8-ounces) black pitted whole olives, drained

2 cups fresh sliced button mushrooms or 1 can (8-ounces) sliced mushrooms, drained and rinsed

1 pound fresh chopped tomatoes or 1 can (14.5-ounces) chopped tomatoes with liquid

1 Tbsp. rice wine vinegar

1/4 grated parmesan or romano cheese

In a large sauté pan, place oil, garlic and onion.

Heat over medium until onion and garlic are mildly cooked.

Add ginger, oregano, and basil. Mix in broccoli, olives, mushrooms, and tomatoes.

Cover and simmer over medium heat until vegetables are tender, but not overdone (about 5 to 10 minutes).

Add vinegar and toss into vegetables. Place into serving dish. Top with grated cheese. Makes 6 servings.

Per serving: 130 Calories, 7 gm PRO, 15 gm CHO, 6 gm FAT, 4 mg Chol, 5 gm Fiber, 416 mg Sodium, 594 mg Potassium.

Green Tea Rice

This recipe has no added fat. If you find it dry, add a drizzle of some canola or olive oil right before serving.

1 cup uncooked rice (I suggest a blend of white, brown and wild rice to provide color, flavor, and fiber)

2 cups water

1 individual serving bag of green tea

1/4 tsp. dried basil*

1/4 tsp. dried oregano*

*Or herbs of your choice

In 3 quart saucepan, boil water and add tea bag. Add rice and herbs.

Reduce heat, cover and simmer on low heat for 20 to 30 minutes (or according to package directions) until cooked.

Remove tea bag prior to serving. Makes 4 servings.

Per serving (without added fat): 170 calories, 4 gm PRO, 36 gm CHO, 1 gm FAT, 0 mg Chol, 2 gm Fiber, 5 mg Sodium (no added salt in analysis), 103 mg Potassium.

Cardiovascular Disease

As defined by the American Heart Association(AHA), cardio-vascular disease (CVD) is a condition that affects the heart and blood vessels.[62,63] It encompasses a number of conditions including coronary artery disease, hypertension (high blood pressure), heart attack, stroke, and angina (chest pain).[64] In the United States it remains a serious health problem.

Coronary Artery Disease (CAD) is a disease caused by narrow-ing of the coronary arteries.[65] The coronary arteries carry blood to the heart. When they become clogged with fat and/or cholesterol deposits, atherosclerosis occurs (think of your water pipes at home and how they become clogged with mineral deposits). This condition causes interference in supplying blood to the heart. When the blood supply is reduced to the heart, chest pain or angina can occur. When the blood supply is blocked by a blood clot in the arteries, a heart attack can occur. The result of a heart attack can be damaging to the heart muscle by depriving it of blood and oxygen; another consequence is death. CAD is the leading cause of death in men and women in the United States.[66]

Cardiovascular disease has risk factors. Some we can change and some we cannot.

What are the major risk factors that *can't* be changed?[67,68]

- **Heredity**—Genetics plays a role in cardiovascular disease.
- **Gender**—Men have a higher risk of having a heart attack; however women catch up after menopause.
- **Increasing age**—Typically over 65 is when the occurrence and death from heart attack increases.

What are the risk factors that *can* be changed?[69,70]

- **High Blood Cholesterol**—Cholesterol is a waxy substance produced by the body. It is necessary in cell membrane function, hormonal synthesis, and nerve insulation. It is also present in animal products. Since our bodies produce it, we don't really "need" to consume it, however what would life be like without it? If we consume a diet high in saturated fats and cholesterol, our blood cholesterol levels will likely rise. As blood cholesterol levels rise, so does the risk of heart attack due to clogged arteries.[71,72] Because elevated cholesterol does not have symptoms, it is important to know your numbers!

A lipid profile is a blood test performed after fasting for a period of time (usually overnight). This profile will provide information such as Total Cholesterol (TC), High Density Lipoprotein (HDL), Low Density Lipoprotein (LDL), and Triglyceride (TG) levels. HDL is known as the lipoprotein which helps carry cholesterol out of your body. LDL is the lipoprotein that sticks to the walls of your arteries and can cause cholesterol buildup— which is not good.[73]

If you have elevated levels of blood fats, your healthcare practitioner should discuss strategies to reduce these levels. Cholesterol levels are measured in milligrams (mg) of cholesterol per deciliter (dL) of blood. See how your cholesterol numbers compare to the tables below.

Total Cholesterol Level	Total Cholesterol Category
Less than 200 mg/dL	Desirable
200–239 mg/dL	Borderline high
240 mg/dL and above	High
LDL Cholesterol Level	**LDL Cholesterol Category**
Less than 100 mg/dL	Optimal
100–129 mg/dL	Near optimal/above optimal
130–159 mg/dL	Borderline high
160–189 mg/dL	High
190 mg/dL and above	Very high
HDL Cholesterol Level	**HDL Cholesterol Category**
Less than 40 mg/dL	A major risk factor for heart disease
40–59 mg/dL	The higher, the better
60 mg/dL and above	Considered protective against heart disease

Reprinted with permission from National Heart Lung and Blood Institute, 2010.
http://www.nhlbi.nih.gov/health/dci/Diseases/Hbc/HBC_Diagnosis.html

High cholesterol can be caused by a number of factors. These include:

- **Diet**—a diet high in saturated fat and cholesterol can increase cholesterol levels. When it comes to diet, the American Heart Association and National Heart Lung and Blood Institute (NHLBI) recommend a diet low in saturated fat and cholesterol (see Fats section, Chapter 6).[74,75] Foods that have been shown to help reduce cholesterol levels include soluble fibers and plant sterols (see Fats and Fiber section, Chapter 6).
- **Body Weight**[76,77]—for some people being overweight and/or obese can elevate cholesterol levels. Reducing weight has been shown to reduce cholesterol while also raising HDL levels and lowering LDL levels.
- **Physical Activity**—regular exercise has been shown to increase HDL levels, and lower LDL levels. Aim for a goal of 30 minutes a day just about every day.
- **Age**—as we age, blood cholesterol levels tend to rise. Women usually have lower total cholesterol numbers levels than men prior to menopause. After menopause, LDL levels tend to rise.
- **Heredity**—Elevated blood lipids can be inherited.
- **Triglycerides**—Triglycerides can also raise your risk for heart disease.[78] Triglycerides (TG) are a form of fat found in our bodies and foods. If you have levels that are borderline high (150 to 199 mg/dL) or high (200 mg/dL or more), your healthcare practitioner may prescribe medication along with a review of diet and lifestyle. Individuals with high TG levels will likely be advised to limit intake of concentrated sweets such as candy, beverages sweetened with sugar, corn syrup, or fructose, simple carbohydrates, and alcohol. In some cases this

condition may be inherited. Below are a few charts with numbers for you to refer. Things that can increase triglyceride levels include:

- Overweight
- Physical inactivity
- Cigarette smoking
- Excessive alcohol use
- Very high carbohydrate diet
- Certain diseases and drugs
- Genetic disorders

Reprinted with permission from National Heart Lung and Blood Institute, 2008. *www.nhlbi.nih.gov/health/dci/Diseases/Hbc/HBC_Diagnosis.html*

Other Cardiovascular Risk Factors That Can be Changed

- **High Blood Pressure**—Elevated blood pressure increases the risk of heart disease and stroke (see section regarding High Blood Pressure in this chapter).[79,80]
- **Smoking**—Smoking can double the risk of a heart attack. It can also increase the likelihood of developing coronary heart disease. It is one of the most addictive and difficult habits to quit. There are many resources out there to help quit smoking. If you smoke, quit! Once you do, within a few years your body can repair itself, and risks are lowered. A few resources include your healthcare practitioner, The American Heart Association (*www.americanheart.org*) The American Cancer Society (*www.cancer.org* or *www.cancer.gov*), The American Lung Association (*www.lungusa.org*), to name a few.
- **Substance Abuse**—Cocaine, alcohol, and other substance abuse can lead to a greater risk of heart disease.[81]

- **Obesity**—Excess weight puts more stress and strain on the heart and arteries. It can also lead to elevated blood cholesterol and diabetes.
- **Physical inactivity**—Exercise can help lower blood pressure, blood cholesterol, body weight, decrease stress, and just make us feel better. Any type of movement in moderation can be of benefit.
- **Stress**—Evidence suggests that chronic stress can lead to greater risk of heart disease. We can learn to handle stress. The majority of us experience stress on a daily basis. The key is dealing with it in a *healthy* manner to take control of it.
- **Control Diabetes/Blood Sugar**—Maintaining healthy blood sugar (glucose) levels and keeping on top of diabetes is important. Elevated blood sugar levels can lead to heart complications and elevated blood lipids.
- **C-reactive protein**—C-reactive protein (CRP) is produced in the liver. Its levels can be raised when there is systemic inflammation in the body. Levels of CRP can be increased in those with cancer, heart attack, irritable bowel syndrome, lupus, rheumatoid arthritis, tuberculosis, or vasculitis. In regards to cardiovascular disease a test performed called a high-sensitivity CRP (hs-CRP) assay can be performed. It is similar to a blood test. This test can determine a person's risk for heart disease. It is considered that an elevated CRP level may be a positive risk factor for cardiovascular disease. However, what it not clear is whether elevated CRP levels are an indicator of, or play an actual part in, heart problems.[82-84]
- **Homocysteine**—an amino acid which has been linked as an independent risk factor for cardiovascular disease. Elevated levels have been linked to an increase in arterial

plaque formation. Dietary intake and genetics both play a part in homocysteine levels. Evidence reveals that a low intake of B vitamins, such as folic acid, B6 and B12 may lower plasma levels of homocysteine. The benefit of lowering homocysteine in relation to reducing risk of cardiovascular disease is still lacking. However, some research suggests that low levels of folic acid are associated with an increased risk of stroke and coronary heart disease.[85,86] Folic acid is found in citrus, asparagus, strawberries, melons, eggs, liver, dark green leafy vegetables, lentils, dried beans, peanuts, avocadoes, and fortified grains. Daily Recommended Intake (DRI) for folic acid is 400 µg. B6 (pyridoxine) is found in chicken, pork, bananas, avocadoes, dried beans, and fortified foods. DRI for B6 is 1.3mg for males and females from age 31 to 50; 50 and beyond is 1.5 mg for females and 1.7 mg for males. As we age, the ability to absorb many nutrients declines, and B12 in particular can be a challenge. B12 (cobalamin) is found primarily in animal products, such as dairy, meats, salmon, shrimp, eggs, poultry, and fortified foods. DRI for B12 is 2.4 µg. Consuming adequate B vitamins may prove to be an ally in heart health.[87]

- **Sleep Apnea**—Sleep apnea is a condition where breathing stops or gets very shallow while sleeping. Left untreated, it can potentially lead to an increased risk in developing high blood pressure, diabetes, heart attack or stroke.[88]

For additional assistance the National Heart Lung and Blood Institute website is *www.nhlbi.nih.gov* and American Heart Association website is *www.americanheart.org*, or you can call your local affiliate for more information.

Recipes

Recipe Acronyms: PRO = Protein; CHO = Carbohydrate; FAT = Fat; Chol =Cholesterol; Gram = gm

Heart Healthy Tuna Tapenade

Enjoy this with crackers, raw vegetables, lettuce leaves, in a sandwich or wrap.

1 can (6-ounces) tuna in water, drained

1 small can (2.25-ounces) pitted black olives, drained

1 garlic clove, peeled

2 tsp. fresh minced rosemary (or 1 tsp. dried)

1 Tbsp. lemon juice

1/4 tsp. black or cayenne pepper (or chile pepper, if you like a little more heat)

1/2 tsp. ground turmeric

2 Tbsp. olive oil

Place everything but the olive oil in a food processor (or mix well by hand) and pulse until blended. Add the olive oil and blend until a paste is formed. Refrigerate. Makes about 1-1/2 cups.

Per 1/4 cup serving: 85 Calories, 7 gm PRO, 6 gm FAT, 1 gm Fiber, 12 mg Chol, 208 mg Sodium, 69 mg Potassium.

Grape Toss

Grapes are an excellent, heart healthy fruit making a great snack alone or as a side dish, salad, or dessert as below.

1/2 lb. green seedless grapes, washed and patted dry (sliced in half, optional), preferably organic

1/2 lb. red or purple seedless grapes, washed and patted dry (sliced in half, optional), preferably organic

1/2 cup chopped walnuts

1/2 cup crumbled blue cheese

1 to 2 Tbsp. balsamic vinegar

1 Tbsp. fresh chopped or 1-2 tsp. dried basil

In a large bowl, mix all ingredients. Start with 1 Tbsp. vinegar and 1 tsp. basil.

Add more according to taste.

Chill for an hour or so. Makes about 6 one-cup servings.

Per serving: 165 Calories, 5 gm PRO, 17 gm CHO, 10 gm FAT, 8 mg Chol, 1.5 gm Fiber, 159 mg Sodium, 248 mg Potassium.

Celiac Disease

Celiac disease, also known as *nontropical sprue*, or gluten sensitive *enteropathy*, is a condition in which individuals cannot tolerate a protein called gluten. Gluten is present in some grains.

Celiac disease is known to be an inherited autoimmune disease that affects 1 in 100 people worldwide.[89] It may also be triggered and occur after surgery, pregnancy, childbirth, emotional stress or a viral infection.

Symptoms are variable and can include gas/bloating, abdominal cramps, diarrhea, constipation, vomiting, muscle cramps, weight loss/gain to name a few. Some individuals may exhibit few, if any symptoms. These can occur at any stage of life.

It is estimated that only 5 to 10 percent of people with celiac disease are diagnosed. Many are misdiagnosed with other conditions, such as Irritable Bowel Syndrome (IBS), chronic fatigue, ulcers, reflux disease and fibromyalgia.[90]

For those with celiac disease, consuming gluten can damage the lining of the small intestine. The result is malabsorption. Consequences of malabsorption include malnutrition, anemia, and osteoporosis. And, because it is an autoimmune disease, it can attack the body systemically and affect other organs, including skin. Infertility in males and females has also been linked with celiac disease.[91-94]

Since many individuals do not elicit actual symptoms, many healthcare practitioners do not test for it. To diagnose celiac disease, blood tests can be performed to detect if an individual has certain antibodies indicating celiac disease may be present. A biopsy of the small intestine is the gold standard to confirm the condition is present.[95-97] When testing is going to occur, it is important to consume gluten containing foods to receive a correct diagnosis.

Gluten is found in barley, rye, and wheat.[98-101] Oats do not naturally contain gluten, however cross contamination can occur during growth, harvesting, processing or transportation. Pure uncontaminated oats are available. A few companies include:

- Bob's Red Mill (*www.bobsredmill.com*)
- Cream Hill Estates (Lara's Brand) (*www.creamhillestates.com*)
- Avena Foods (*www.onlyoats.com*)
- Gifts of Nature (*www.giftsofnature.net*)
- Gluten-Free Oats (*www.glutenfreeoats.com*)

In most cases, small to moderate amounts of oats are tolerated in those with celiac disease. However, a small population may not tolerate pure oats.[102]

The treatment for celiac disease is a lifelong gluten free diet. Symptoms may improve within a few weeks, however, and the intestines may take six months to two years for the villi to be healed. Staying on this regimen is for life, as eating gluten containing products will start the damage all over again.[103-106] Drugs that may block the reaction to gluten are currently being researched, and may someday allow for those with gluten sensitivity/intolerance to consume small quantities.[107]

Following a gluten free diet can be challenging. In addition to the obvious gluten containing products such as breads, cakes, cookies, crackers, cereals and pasta, it is found in a wide variety of foods, beverages, some medications, supplements, and lip balms.[108,109] Some of these include:

- Processed meats, sauces, salad dressings, gravies, seasonings
- Soups
- Flavored coffees and teas
- Candy
- Communion wafers
- Cake frosting
- Seasoned potato chips and nuts
- Imitation fish products
- Canned baked beans
- Malt, malt flavoring, extract
- Hydrolyzed wheat protein
- Wheat flour, wheat starch
- Beer, ale and lager

Check the label and look for products that state they are Gluten Free.[110]

The good news is there are a number of gluten free products available, ranging from baked goods, cereals, snack bars, soups, condiments, and gluten free beer.[111] They can be considerably more expensive to purchase, however.[112]

Gluten free grains and flours to utilize in cooking include amaranth, corn, buckwheat, millet, potato, rice, sorghum, soy, tapioca. Millet, rice, quinoa and buckwheat can be utilized in place of wheat, rye and barley. Unprocessed fruits, vegetables, plain meats, seafood, poultry, pork, nuts, legumes, eggs, milk and cheese can all be included in a gluten free diet.[113,114]

Sometimes those with celiac disease may have a temporary lactose intolerance due to the damaged villi in the intestine from inflammation. There are lactose free dairy products and a supplement called Lact-aid® that can assist in digestion and absorption of dairy. It is important to consider utilizing these products to maintain calcium intake for bone and immune health.

If a person continues to consume gluten, conditions such as malnutrition, anemia, autoimmune disease, thyroid disease, and lymphoma may occur. Thus it is important to be checked for this condition.

It is important to work with a registered dietitian experienced with celiac disease to assist you in learning about the condition and throughout the process of adjusting your food intakes. In helping you follow a gluten free diet successfully, a registered dietitian can be found at *www.eatright.org*. Look for a nutrition professional in your local area. Additional resources include *www.glutenfreediet.ca*, *www.savorypalate.com*, *www.celiac.org*, *www.gluten.net*, *www.celiac.ca*, and *www.digestive.niddk.nih.gov/ddiseases/pubs/celiac/#1*. When travelling or dining out, refer to *www.glutenfreepassport.com* as well as *www.triumphdining.com*, and, when in Canada, *www.theceliacscene.com*.

Recipes

Recipe Acronyms: PRO = Protein; CHO = Carbohydrate;
FAT = Fat; Chol = Cholesterol; Gram = gm

The following is a delicious recipe from Carol Fenster:

Carol Fenster's French Bread

Put this bread into a cold oven for a crisp crust and nice texture.
If this doesn't work in your oven, let the bread rise until level with
top of pan; then bake in preheated 425°F oven for 25 to 30
minutes. Use a pan specially designed for French bread.

2 Tbsp. active dry yeast

1-1/4 cups warm (110°F) milk of choice

1 Tbsp. sugar

2 cups Carol's Sorghum Blend (see below)

1 cup potato starch

1 tsp. xanthan gum

1 tsp. guar gum

1/4 cup nonfat dry milk powder (not Carnation) or Better Than
Milk soy powder

1-1/4 tsp. salt

1 Tbsp. butter or buttery spread, softened

3 large egg whites

1 tsp. cider vinegar

Egg wash (optional—1 egg white, beaten with 1 Tbsp. water)

Dissolve sugar and yeast in warm water. Set aside for 5 minutes.
Grease French bread pans or line with parchment paper.

In bowl of heavy-duty stand mixer, combine all ingredients
(sorghum blend through vinegar) plus yeast-milk mixture. Beat
on low speed to blend, then beat on medium speed for 30
seconds, scraping down sides with spatula. Dough will be soft.

166

Divide dough in half on prepared pan. Smooth each half into 12-inch log with wet spatula. Brush with egg wash for glossier crust. Make 3 diagonal slashes (1/8-inch deep) in each loaf so steam can escape during rising.

Place immediately on middle rack in cold oven. Set to 425°F oven and bake approximately 30 to 35 minutes, or until nicely browned.

Remove bread from pans; cool completely on wire rack before slicing with electric knife. Makes 2 loaves. Serves 20 (1-inch slices).

Per serving: 83 calories, 2 gm PRO, 17gm CHO, 1 gm FAT, 2 mg Chol, 1 gm Fiber, 159 mg Sodium.

Carol's Sorghum Blend

1-1/2 cups sorghum flour

1-1/2 cups potato starch

1 cup tapioca

Whisk together and store, tightly covered, in a dark, dry place.

Reprinted with permission from Carol Fenster *www.savorypalate.com*, author of Gluten Free 101 (Wiley).

Dental Hygiene

Our teeth are more than just for chewing and a nice smile. While taking care of your teeth can help reduce the occurrence of cavities and gum disease, good dental hygiene can play a role in overall health.

Did you know that poor dental health has also been linked to conditions such as heart disease, stroke, premature low weight births, respiratory infections, arthritis, memory impairment, and oral infections with diabetes?[115,116]

Developing a routine of oral hygiene is like any other habit. It takes some time, but once established it can be easy to follow. Here are a few tips:

What You Can Do to Maintain Good Oral Health

- **Discuss fluoride with your healthcare practitioner/ dentist.** Fluoride has been shown to help prevent tooth decay; excess may affect bone health later in life.
- **Take care of your teeth and gums.** Thorough tooth brushing and flossing to reduce dental plaque can prevent gingivitis—the mildest form of gum disease.
- **Avoid tobacco.** In addition to the general health risks posed by tobacco, smokers have four times the risk of developing gum disease compared to non-smokers. Tobacco use in any form—cigarette, pipes, and smokeless (spit) tobacco—increases the risk for gum disease, oral and throat cancers, and oral fungal infection (candidiasis). Spit tobacco containing sugar increases the risk of tooth decay. Additional information is available at *www.cdc.gov/nccdphp/publications/CDNR/.*
- **Limit alcohol.** Heavy use of alcohol is also a risk factor for oral and throat cancers. When used alone, alcohol and tobacco are risk factors for oral cancers, but when used in combination the effects of alcohol and tobacco are even greater.
- **Eat wisely.** Adults should limit snacks full of sugars and starches. The recommended five-a-day helping of fiber-rich fruits and vegetables stimulates salivary flow to aid remineralization of tooth surfaces with early stages of tooth decay.
- **Visit the dentist regularly.** Check-ups can detect early signs of oral health problems and can lead to treatments that will prevent further damage, and in some cases,

reverse the problem. Professional tooth cleaning (prophylaxis) also is important for preventing oral problems, especially when self-care is difficult.

- **Diabetic patients should work to maintain control of their health.** This will help prevent the complications of diabetes, including an increased risk of gum disease.
- **If medications produce a dry mouth, ask your doctor if there are other drugs that can be substituted.** If dry mouth cannot be avoided, drink plenty of water, chew sugarless gum, and avoid tobacco and alcohol.
- **Have an oral health check-up before beginning cancer treatment.** Radiation to the head or neck and/or chemotherapy may cause problems for your teeth and gums. Treating existing oral health problems before cancer therapy may help prevent or limit oral complications or tissue damage.

Above reprinted with permission from
www.cdc.gov/oralhealth/publications/factsheets/adult.htm

Foods we eat can have an impact on our teeth. Every time we eat, acids are formed in the mouth to assist with digestion. These acids can start the process of tooth decay if not treated.[117] In addition to the above suggestions there are certain foods that have been linked with helping to keep a healthier mouth. These include:

- Foods rich in calcium and phosphorus such as sugar free dairy products, poultry, meats and nuts.
- Green tea. Green tea has been shown to help reduce the growth of bacteria in the mouth. One study revealed that one to two cups per day reduced tooth loss risk by 18 percent.[118]
- Unsweetened beverages.

- Crispy fruits and vegetables, which as mentioned above can stimulate saliva production.
- If consuming simple sugars, starches, or acidic foods such as tomato or citrus products, try to incorporate them into a meal and consume water or a sugar free beverage to help rinse the mouth.
- Chew sugarless gum, especially after meals or sugary/starchy snacks. Sugarless gum can help clean teeth out. Be careful if you have jaw problems, however.[119]
- Omega-3 fatty acids. Research conducted on the anti-bacterial effects of omega-3 fatty acids looked promising in a study published in *Molecular Oral Microbiology* in regards to reducing the growth of oral pathogens.[120,121]

Diabetes

Diabetes is a disease in which the body does not produce or utilize insulin efficiently.[122-124] Insulin is a hormone secreted by the pancreas. It is the key that lets glucose into the cell to be metabolized for energy. Glucose is produced by the foods we eat (primarily carbohydrates). Insulin also helps in the metabolism of amino acids (protein) and fatty acids (fats). Hyperglycemia (high blood sugar) is a characteristic of diabetes. It is a metabolic disease that affects the body from head to toe—literally. Elevated blood sugar levels can wreak havoc on our bodies over the long term. A few examples include:

- Increase in infections, such as yeast or urinary tract
- Vision loss
- Wound healing
- Elevated blood lipid levels
- Diminished kidney function and damage
- Impaired nerve function and damage

- Circulatory problems
- Loss of limbs

Diabetes is a major risk factor for heart attack and stroke.[125-128] Some people may have diabetes and don't even know it. A few symptoms include blurred vision, unexplained weakness or fatigue, irritability, frequent urination, extreme hunger or thirst, weight loss and sores that don't heal.[129-133]

Your healthcare practitioner can perform a few simple tests to see if you have a high blood sugar, and potentially diabetes. One test is called Fasting Plasma Glucose Test (FPG). Blood is drawn after an individual has not eaten for at least 8 hours. If the fasting blood glucose is between 100 to 125 mg/dl, this is known as *pre-diabetes*. In pre-diabetes, blood glucose levels are elevated but not high enough for a diagnosis of diabetes. If the blood glucose level is 126 mg/dl or above, that is considered diabetes.[134]

Another test is called an Oral Glucose Tolerance Test (OGTT). This fasting glucose test involves measuring the blood glucose level after a person has fasted at least 8 hours and two hours after ingesting a glucose rich beverage. If the two-hour blood glucose level is between 140 and 199 mg/dl, that is considered pre-diabetes. If the two-hour blood glucose measures 200 mg/dl or higher, then the individual has diabetes.[135]

Another blood test your healthcare practitioner may perform is a random plasma glucose test, also called a casual plasma glucose test. The test measures blood glucose without regard to when the person being tested last ate. This test, along with an assessment of symptoms, is used to diagnose diabetes but not pre-diabetes.[136] There are three types of diabetes: **Type 1**, **Type 2**, and **Gestational**.

Type 1 Diabetes

It is a condition in which the body does not produce insulin. It is an autoimmune disease.[137,138] An autoimmune disease is when the body starts attacking itself. In this case, the pancreatic beta cells are the ones attacked. The pancreatic beta cells produce insulin. Since these cells are attacked and thus destroyed, the body is no longer able to produce insulin.

It is thought that the development of an autoimmune response to a virus can precipitate Type 1 diabetes in those that are susceptible. It can be an inherited or genetically predisposed condition. It is usually diagnosed in children and young adults, but some adults may be diagnosed as well.

Type 1 diabetes is more common in colder climates; it is also less common in those who were breastfed.[139]

Management of blood glucose is a necessary part of this condition. It is necessary to inject insulin daily or utilize an insulin pump (and maybe someday inhale insulin) to assist with the proper absorption of glucose.[140,141] Understanding how foods, activity level, stress, medications, herbs, etc., affect an individual's blood glucose level is important to managing insulin levels.[142-144]

Most diabetics keep a log of their blood glucose levels. Similar to keeping a journal of food, activity and stress, these logs can help assess what may affect blood glucose levels in both types of diabetes. Maintaining consistency is key in managing Type 1 diabetes.

Type 2 Diabetes

Type 2 diabetes is the more common form of diabetes. It is mainly a result of the body either not producing enough insulin or having insulin resistance. Many times it can be managed by diet, exercise, and in some cases, medication. Many people are able to control it by losing or managing their body weight and incorporating exercise to increase insulin sensitivity. It too, can be hereditary. Some factors found to increase the risk of Type 2 diabetes are excess body weight, physical inactivity, high saturated and trans fat intake, consumption of simple sugars and alcohol, along with low fiber intake.[145,146]

The incidence of Type 2 diabetes continues to rise in the United States. Is it any coincidence considering that food portion sizes have increased and our physical activity has decreased? What is happening is that when we eat more calories than we need, blood sugar levels tend to rise. The body can only metabolize so much at a time. Think of it as if you put too much gasoline in your car—it would overflow. The difference with your body is that the extra glucose stays circulating in the bloodstream and manifests itself in different ways as mentioned earlier. For those who are at risk of developing Type 2 diabetes, a change in diet and lifestyle with as little as a 5 percent reduction in excess weight can possibly help alleviate the need for medication.[147]

Much of the treatment of diabetes relies upon maintenance of blood sugar levels, along with diet and lifestyle choices. Typically, such a regimen includes monitoring blood sugar, incorporating exercise, managing stress, maintaining oral hygiene and understanding what influence foods have on the body. Eating throughout the day is essential in order to control blood sugar and assist in the utilization of medication.[148-150] Complex carbohydrates and high fiber foods play a role in maintaining blood glucose levels.[151,152]

Other compounds have been shown to assist in the risk reduction and treatment of diabetes. Individuals who consume higher levels of magnesium have been shown to have a reduced risk of developing diabetes. Magnesium assists in the utilization and metabolism of insulin. In the processing of foods, magnesium is one of the minerals that may not make it back into the original product. Thus, many individuals are likely consuming less magnesium. Food sources of magnesium include almonds, buckwheat, shredded wheat, cooked spinach, potatoes, plain yogurt, milk, brown rice, whole wheat bread, salmon, and bananas. The Daily Recommended Intake (DRI) for magnesium is 420 mg for men; 320 mg for women.[153]

Chromium is another mineral that has been shown to help in the metabolism of glucose by turning it into energy. As it may enhance removal of glucose from the blood, chromium may also be of benefit to those with Type 2 diabetes. Sources of chromium include brewer's yeast, egg yolks, meats, liver, potatoes (with the skins), cheeses, molasses, whole grain breads and cereals, and fresh fruits and vegetables. Keep in mind, too much chromium (usually via supplements) can lead to stomach disturbance, low blood sugar, damage to the liver, kidneys, nerves, and cause irregular heart rhythm.[154-158]

The United States Department of Agriculture (USDA) estimates a DRI of 25mcg/day for women 31 to 50 and 20 mcg/day for women 50 and over; 35 mcg/day for men 31 to 50 and 30 mcg/day for men 51 and up.[159]

For those with Type 2 diabetes some studies have shown that supplementation with divided doses of chromium picolinate ranging from 200 to 1000 mcg/day may improve glucose and insulin uptake.[160-163]

Portion sizes are very important in a diabetic's regimen, as these can determine what effect they will have on blood sugar. So is the quality of the food. It is also imperative that someone with diabetes take care of their body early on. Having regular eye examinations, physical examinations, taking care of feet, skin, teeth and full body is essential in managing this condition. Many diabetics I have counseled over the years with diabetes exhibited no symptoms in the early years of the disease. Then, all of a sudden, eye problems, circulatory problems, chronic infections, wounds that took a long time to heal, etc., were occurring on a regular basis. Another difficulty I faced in the past when counseling individuals was finding what foods would fit into their particular lifestyle. It was (and is) not realistic to hand someone a pre-printed diet sheet with foods they were not going to eat. Many factors need consideration—age, sex, activity level, economics, culture, religion, and health status all need to be part of the plan. Some of what I call the "high riser's" of blood sugar are simple carbohydrates (see Carbohydrate section, Chapter 6). These are foods which have a nasty habit of raising the blood sugar levels. They also raise triglycerides, lower the good guy fats such as HDL, and increase inflammatory factors in the blood.

Gestational Diabetes

Gestational diabetes occurs during the latter part of pregnancy. It is a temporary condition. Women with a family history of Type 2 diabetes, overweight/obese women, and those over forty are at higher risk of developing gestational diabetes. Hormonal changes during pregnancy are the primary cause.

High blood pressure and toxemia (swelling, high blood pressure and excess protein in the urine) are at increased risk in women with gestational diabetes. It does need to be monitored during pregnancy. It usually disappears after giving birth. However, some women who develop gestational diabetes are at risk for developing Type 2 diabetes later in life.[164-166]

The American Diabetes website is *www.diabetes.org*, or you can call your local affiliate for more information.

Since we are discussing the endocrine system, it might be worth noting that many folks who enter their menopausal years may find they become sluggish and gain weight. There's a chance it could be your thyroid. Check with your healthcare practitioner.

Things Not Sweet Enough for You?

Many diabetics use sugar substitutes instead of table sugar. These products can substitute the taste of sugar without raising blood glucose or insulin levels. Another benefit they offer is a reduction in dental caries. There is a variety on the market these days. They include aspartame, acesulfame-K, saccharin, sucralose, sorbitol, mannitol, xylitol and stevia to name a few.[167]

The way artificial sweeteners work is they are metabolized like a sugar but at a slower rate, which is why they do not raise blood glucose like simple sugars. Sugar alcohols such as sorbitol, mannitol, and xylitol can also cause some gastric upset and have a laxative effect if consumed in large quantities.[168] A number of sugar free candies and some baked goods are made with these products. There is usually an indication on the package of these type of products indicating possible side effects.

On a more natural note, one compound in the spice rack scientists are finding of benefit is cinnamon.[169-171] It has been shown to improve the metabolism of glucose, along with lowering blood pressure and cholesterol. About 1/4 tsp. per day is what has been studied.[172] Cinnamon contains antioxidants called polyphenols.[173] Polyphenols have been shown to reduce inflammation. While more research is being performed, adding a little cinnamon (without sugar) has not been shown to be harmful, and it adds flavor. Again, keep in mind a little may go a long way. Too much of anything may not provide any added benefit. Cinnamon can be added to everything from coffee, cereal, on toast, in casseroles, sauces, etc. But, keep in mind, cinnamon does have the potential to interact with medications or supplements.

Cardiovascular disease and diabetes are closely linked, because they both involve circulation. As mentioned in the Cardiovascular Disease section in this chapter, think of your arteries like your plumbing. Mineral deposits and goo will clog the pipes. Same goes for your arteries. The liquid plumber foods are things we have reviewed such as:

- Omega-3 fats
- Olive and canola oils
- Raw garlic
- Oatmeal
- Nuts (preferably unsalted)
- Whole grains
- Flaxseed
- Colorful foods like berries, tomatoes, red peppers, spinach, greens, herbs like cilantro and parsley, spices like ginger, turmeric

Having a high carbohydrate meal? Request vinegar (and if need be some olive oil) for your salad and bread. Vinegar has been shown to help regulate blood glucose/sugar levels so they won't spike as high.[174] Every little bit helps ...

Recipes

Recipe Acronyms: PRO = Protein; CHO = Carbohydrate; FAT = Fat; Chol = Cholesterol; Gram = gm

Beans are a high fiber and heart healthy soluble fiber food that can help control blood sugar. The darker the color of the bean, the more antioxidants it contains. This recipe is a fast and economical way to enjoy a satisfying meal.

Easy Beans and Rice

1 can (15-ounces) no added salt black or red beans, rinsed and drained

1 can (12.5-ounces) chopped stewed tomatoes

1/2 cup salsa, optional

1 cup frozen chopped spinach

1/2 tsp. cinnamon

1/2 tsp. dried oregano

2 cups hot cooked rice (brown, preferably or a mixture of brown and white)

1 clove garlic, chopped

In a saucepan, combine beans, oil, tomatoes, salsa (if desired) spinach, and cinnamon.

Add a little water to the pot (about 1/3 to 1/2 cup) so mixture will not scorch.

Cover and simmer until heated.

Remove from heat and stir in hot rice and raw chopped garlic (the potent compounds in garlic are present when it is raw).

Serve. Garnish with cilantro, parsley, salsa, grated cheese, sour cream or plain yogurt, etc. Makes 4 servings.

Per serving: 360 Calories, 19 gm PRO, 70 gm CHO, 2 gm FAT, 19 gm Fiber, 0 mg Chol, 500 mg Sodium, 965 mg Potassium.

EZ Guacamole

1 avocado, washed, peeled, pitted and mashed

Lemon juice (enough to coat avocado to prevent browning— about 1-2 tsp.)

1/4 cup salsa, drained

1/4 tsp. ground cumin, optional

Mix avocado and lemon juice.

Stir in salsa to taste.

Add cumin if desired. Store in covered container and refrigerate for at least 30 minutes. Makes 4 servings.

Per serving: 65 Calories, 1gm PRO, 4 gm CHO, 5.5 gm FAT, 3 gm Fiber, 0 mg Chol, 100 mg Sodium, 232 mg Potassium.

Snack ideas

Go for the complex carbohydrates as they have more fiber and will help maintain blood sugar longer. Also include some protein and fat. Here are a few:

- Hummus with chips/crackers/veggies
- Cottage cheese with fruit or vegetables
- Pretzels with nuts and dried fruit
- Hardboiled egg with crackers, raw veggies
- Veggies with melted cheese (if there's a microwave at work, take it with you to heat up and have some salsa handy)
- Small quesadilla
- Half or whole Sandwich
- Cheese or peanut butter with crackers or fruit
- Glass of instant breakfast drink (there are sugar free varieties)
- One cup of sugar free or plain yogurt with your choice of added goodies such as fruit, cereal, nuts, etc.
- Stir in ground flaxseed to nut butters, spreads, yogurt, and casseroles to bump up the fiber, and add some omega-3 fatty acids.

Eye Health

Do you have to hold reading material a little farther away to be able to read it? Many of us start to experience changes in our vision in our late 30s to early 40s. It is estimated that one in three Americans will develop some form of vision-impairing eye disease by age 65.[175]

Additional age-related eye changes that occur in midlife include cataracts, dry eye, and age-related macular degeneration. Vision may not be affected by these conditions initially. The American Academy of Opthalmology recommends getting a baseline eye exam around age 40.[176]

Let's review these conditions and learn how to keep our eyes healthy.

Cataracts

A normal eye lens, which is made up of mostly protein and water, is transparent and allows for light to refract and focus on the retina which allows for a clear image.[177-178] When the protein clumps up, it clouds the lens and reduces the amount of light into the eye. A cataract is a clouding of the lens of the eye which impairs vision.[179-181]

Cataracts develop gradually. While many think it is part of aging, lifestyle factors such as smoking, unprotected exposure to ultraviolet light (UV) sunlight, and a diet low in antioxidants may all play a part in the development of cataracts. Additional factors include family history, diabetes, being overweight and long term use of steroids and beta blockers.[182-186] One study showed that elderly individuals with heart disease who took antidepressants (SSRI's) showed a greater risk of developing cataracts.[187]

Most people have their cataracts surgically removed. It is typically a simple procedure and results are usually immediate.[188,189]

What to do to slow it down:

- Wear protective sunglasses and a wide brim hat to protect your eyes from UV sunlight exposure.
- Stop smoking.

- Manage weight.
- Control blood sugar, meaning ditch the simple carbohydrates.
- Eat plenty of antioxidant rich foods, including dark green leafy vegetables, green tea, and others discussed in the Antioxidants section (Chapter 3) of this book.[190-194] A Harvard study showed that women who consumed a regular diet of fruits and vegetables had a 10 to 15 percent less chance of developing cataracts. High blood levels of vitamin C (found in citrus, broccoli, peppers, kiwi, berries) reduced cataract development; omega-3 fatty acids also lowered cataract risk in a Tufts University study of women.[195]

Dry Eye

Dry eye has a number of causes. It can be temporary or chronic. A few include:

- Hormonal changes with menopause, which is why women tend to have a higher incidence
- Use of medications, including antihistamines, nasal decongestants, tranquilizers, blood pressure medications, birth control pills, Parkinson's medications, antidepressants
- Skin disease on or around the eyelid
- Pregnancy
- Women taking hormone replacement therapy
- Allergies
- LASIK surgery—the effect may be short term, such as three to six months, but may last longer
- Inadequate blinking, especially when staring at a computer or video screen
- Inadequate or excessive dosages of vitamins

- Autoimmune disorders such as Sjogren's, rheumatoid arthritis, or collagen vascular diseases
- Use of contact lenses[196-199]

Dry eye is treated on an individual basis. Some treatments include prescription and non-prescription eye drops, surgical procedures, temporary or permanent closure of the tear ducts. Omega-3 fatty acids have been shown to help improve dry eye.[200,201] Eating a healthy diet that provides essential vitamins and minerals for eye health is very important. These include lutein, zeaxanthin, vitamin C, E (not more than 100 percent of vitamin E), and beta carotene.[202] It is important to review eating, medication and use of supplements with your healthcare practitioner and discuss your dietary intake with a registered dietitian. Wearing sunglasses to protect the eyes is important. When using a computer, video screen or watching television, it is important to remember to blink and look away from the screen every so often.

Age-Related Macular Degeneration

In order to see clearly in order to complete regular tasks we need central vision. The macula is located in the center of the retina, which is the light sensitive tissue at the back of the eye. The retina instantly converts light, or an image, into electrical impulses. The retina then sends these impulses, or nerve signals, to the brain.[203]

Age-related macular degeneration (AMD) is a condition in which the macula of the eye is gradually deteriorated or destroyed. AMD is the leading cause of vision loss in the United States for people over age 60.[204,205] While an individual may not go blind with AMD, vision may become blurred, dark spots may be present and central vision may be distorted or lost. Peripheral (side) vision may be retained with AMD.[206] There are two forms of AMD—wet and dry.

Wet AMD

Wet AMD occurs when abnormal blood vessels behind the retina start to grow under the macula. These new blood vessels tend to be very fragile and often leak blood and fluid. The blood and fluid raise the macula from its normal place at the back of the eye. Scar tissue may also be formed. Damage to the macula occurs rapidly.[207,208]

Dry AMD

Dry AMD occurs when the light-sensitive cells in the macula slowly break down, gradually blurring central vision in the affected eye. It is typically the more common form of AMD. As dry AMD gets worse, you may see a blurred spot in the center of your vision. Over time, as less of the macula functions, central vision is gradually lost in the affected eye.

The most common symptom of dry AMD is slightly blurred vision. You may have difficulty recognizing faces. You may need more light for reading and other tasks. Dry AMD generally affects both eyes, but vision can be lost in one eye while the other eye seems unaffected.[209-211] Those at risk for developing AMD include:

- Individuals over 60—While AMD may develop at middle age, the older we get, the greater the risk of developing AMD.
- Smoking
- Family history
- Gender—Women are more likely to develop AMD.
- Race—Caucasians are more likely to lose vision to AMD than African Americans.

While there is no known cure for AMD, there may be ways to slow the progression of the condition. The National Eye Institute conducted a study called the age-related eye disease study (AREDS). The study was designed to learn more about the natural history and risk factors of age-related macular degeneration (AMD) and cataract formation. An additional goal was to evaluate the effect of high doses of antioxidants and zinc on the progression of AMD and cataracts. Results from the AREDS showed that high levels of antioxidants and zinc significantly reduce the risk of advanced age-related macular degeneration (AMD) and its associated vision loss. These same nutrients however had no significant effect on the development or progression of cataracts. AREDS did show that over a six year period the progression of advanced macular degeneration was reduced by 25 percent by the use of antioxidants zinc and vitamins C, E and beta carotene.

High levels of vitamin E, however are not recommended as they may have the potential to increase inflammation of C-reactive protein, which has also been linked with an increase in risk of developing macular degeneration.[212-215] It is important to note that when considering supplementation, you must discuss it with your healthcare practitioner. As mentioned throughout this book, supplements have interactions with medications and conditions. They are not a one-size-fits-all approach.

The study was so successful there is now an AREDS2 study under way. AREDS2 is a nationwide study to determine whether a modified combination of vitamins, minerals and fish oil can further slow the progression of vision loss. For more information go to *www.nei.nih.gov/news/pressreleases/101206.asp*.

Lifestyle factors to help slow the progression of AMD.[216]

- Stop smoking.
- Manage weight.
- Eat a healthy diet high in dark leafy green vegetables and fish-think antioxidants and plenty of color.

- Lutein and zeaxanthin are found in high concentrations in the macula. Think orange and dark green.[217]
- Eggs are also a good source of lutein, zeaxanthin and zinc.
- Consume foods containing omega-3 fatty acids on a regular basis. Docosahexanoic acid (DHA) is an omega-3 fatty acid. It plays a role in eye health. It is found in fatty fish, algal oil, organ meats and breast milk.[218-221]
- Exercise.
- Maintain normal blood pressure.
- Manage blood sugar; consume complex vs. simple carbohydrates.

Recipes

Recipe Acronyms: PRO = Protein; CHO = Carbohydrate; FAT = Fat; Chol = Cholesterol; Gram = gm

Spinach Basil Pesto

Here's a great (and sneaky) way to get some nutrient rich spinach in a delicious pesto sauce. Pesto can be used in pasta, pizza, on a baked potato, in a tuna or salmon salad, and as a spread on sandwiches and meats. Make up a batch and refrigerate up to a week or freeze up to 6 months. One tip for using smaller quantities—freeze pesto in ice cube trays.

2 cloves garlic, peeled

1/4 cup walnuts

3/4 cup freshly grated parmesan cheese

2 cups fresh spinach, preferably organic, washed and drained

2 cups fresh basil. washed and drained

1/2 cup olive oil

In a food processor or blender, place garlic and blend until well minced.

Add walnuts and parmesan cheese to form a dry paste.

Add spinach and basil and process until blended.

Gradually add olive oil while processor or blender is on.
Makes 2 cups.

Season with salt and pepper as desired, however the parmesan cheese contains salt, so you may not even need to use any.

Per Tablespoon: 50 calories, 1 gm PRO, 5 gm FAT, 2 mg Chol, 35 mg sodium, 196 IU vitamin A, 238 mcg lutein and zeaxanthin, 30 mg calcium, 20 mg potassium, 72 mg omega-3 fatty acids, 0.2 mg zinc

Brussels, Beets, and Sweets

This colorful hearty side dish goes well with beef, pork, game, tofu, turkey or chicken. It's easy to make, full of flavor and loaded with nutrition. Enjoy!

1/4 tsp salt

1/4 tsp. black pepper

1/2 tsp. cinnamon

2 tsp. dried rosemary

3 cloves garlic, minced

2 tsp. minced fresh ginger

1 medium onion, rinsed, peeled and chopped

2 lbs. sweet potatoes, rinsed, scrubbed and cut into bite size chunks

1 lb. beets, rinsed, peeled, and cut into bite size chunks

1/2 lb. fresh or 1 bag (12-ounces) frozen Brussels sprouts, rinsed and cut into halves

2 Tbsp. canola oil

Preheat oven to 400°F.

In small bowl, combine spices, garlic and ginger. Set aside.

On large cookie sheet or baking pan assemble all vegetables.

Drizzle canola oil over vegetables and mix together with tongs (or clean hands).

Sprinkle garlic, ginger, salt, pepper, cinnamon, and rosemary on top of vegetable mixture and stir to coat well.

Bake for 25 minutes. Take out of oven and stir vegetables. Place back into oven and bake another 25 to 30 minutes until cooked. Makes 6 servings.

Per serving: 200 calories, 4 gm PRO, 35 gm CHO, 5 gm FAT, 0 mg Chol, 7 gm Fiber, 227 mg sodium, 789 mg potassium, 16203 IU vitamin A, 39 mg vitamin C, 595 mcg lutein and zeaxanthin, 80 mg omega-3 fatty acids, 0.8 mg zinc

Gastroesophageal Reflux Disease (GERD)

GERD is a condition where the stomach contents or acids back up into the esophagus. Symptoms include:

- Heartburn
- Difficulty swallowing
- Regurgitation
- Sensation of a lump in the throat
- Dry cough
- Hoarseness
- Sinus infections
- Asthma symptoms[222-224]

Factors contributing to the causes of GERD include:

- Hiatal hernia
- Obesity
- Pregnancy
- Smoking

- Diabetes
- Delayed stomach emptying[225-227]

GERD has also been linked to a condition called Barrett's esophagus; this is a condition where the cells in the esophageal lining take on an abnormal shape and can eventually become cancerous.[228,229]

A study in the *New England Journal of Medicine* found that women with increased body weight had an increase in GERD or GERD-like symptoms. And, when weight was reduced, the incidence of GERD was reduced.[230]

As mentioned in the Asthma section, many people can develop asthma related GERD (even many children with asthma could have GERD aggravating their condition). What to do? First, check with your physician or healthcare practitioner. Lifestyle factors to manage GERD include:

- Attaining or maintaining a healthy weight.
- Avoid eating or drinking two to three hours prior to bedtime.
- Stop smoking.
- Avoid foods or beverages that may aggravate symptoms, such as alcohol, coffee, chocolate, tomato products, and citrus.
- Large meals may also increase the likelihood of heartburn and reflux. Consume smaller meals throughout the day.
- For some individuals elevating the head of the bed may help.
- Wear loose fitting clothes.
- There are also a number of medications that can help alleviate symptoms and control the condition and its symptoms.

- If you experience difficulty swallowing, and have frequent heartburn, have it checked.[231-233]

Early detection and treatment can alleviate problems later in life.

Health Note: An important note regarding proton pump inhibitors (PPI's). The role of this class of drugs is to suppress the production of stomach acids. Our bodies were designed to produce stomach acids to aid in digestion. These drugs were also initially designed to take for a short term. Long term use of PPI's can lead to potential nutrition deficiencies including calcium, iron and vitamin B_{12} due to lack of stomach acids. Nutrition deficiencies can lead to other conditions including anemia, depression, hip fractures, and other ailments.[234-236] Discuss this with your healthcare practitioner.

For more information, go to:
National Digestive Diseases Information Clearinghouse at *www.digestive.niddk.nih.gov/ddiseases/pubs/gerd/* or, American Gastroenterological Association, at *www.gastro.org* and click on *patient center.*

High Blood Pressure (Hypertension)

Hypertension has been known as the silent killer throughout the years. There are many people walking around with it, and don't even know they have it. Blood pressure is the force of blood against the walls of the arteries. It is measured by two numbers known as systole(ic) and diastole (ic). Systolic is the pressure when the heart beats (which is the larger number), and diastolic is the pressure when the heart relaxes between beats (which is the smaller number).

A normal blood pressure is around 120/80mmHg (120 is the systolic and 80 is the diastolic). High Blood Pressure occurs when the there is higher than normal pressure on blood vessel walls. Many times it can occur when the artery is damaged, or by plaque build-up from high cholesterol on the walls of arteries. When this pressure is prolonged it increases the workload of the heart, and can contribute to plaque formation in the arteries. This can increase one's risk for developing heart disease, kidney disease, blindness or stroke. The National Heart Lung and Blood Institute (NHLBI) estimates that one in every three American adults has high blood pressure.[237]

To help prevent and control this condition maintaining a healthy lifestyle is the key. Recommendations include consuming a moderate amount salt/sodium, attain/maintain a healthy weight, exercise, quit smoking, watch alcohol intake manage stress, increase fruit, vegetable, and whole grain intake, and consume adequate calcium.[238,239] Also, the Dietary Approaches to Stop Hypertension (DASH) diet is a successful program that has been shown to reduce blood pressure.

In some cases, your physician or healthcare practitioner may recommend medication. Getting REAL (Realistic Eating And Lifestyle) is most likely the prescription your healthcare practitioner will give you.

One of the things you can do to offset some of your sodium intake is to increase your potassium intake. Sodium and potassium are electrolytes that help conduct electrical flow in the body. They also regulate fluid balance, nerve transmission, cell membrane activity, and cardiac muscle function. They act like a symphony together (other electrolytes include calcium and magnesium) working to help keep our bodies humming. If we don't have that balance, we can not only have cardiac problems, but experience mental confusion, fatigue, muscle weakness, dizziness, and thirst.

Salt as we know it is a mixture of sodium chloride. Sodium makes up 40 percent and chloride 60 percent.[240] There are other sources of sodium in our foods. Some are naturally occurring and some are added as a flavoring or preservative agent. Baking soda (sodium bicarbonate) and sodium bisulfite are a few examples. When reading labels, check for sodium in the ingredient section as well as in the content section. For those with hypertension, the American Heart Association recommends a daily intake of 1500 mg or less of sodium. The average American consumes about 3400 mg per day.[241] In some individuals, sodium can cause retention of fluids, aggravating hypertension and putting more work on the heart.

This imbalance is sort of like an orchestra missing an instrument. It doesn't feel or sound right, as something is off. Eating more potassium in your diet can include sources such as:

- Fresh or dried fruits (especially berries, citrus, apricots, melons, bananas, kiwi, mango, plums/prunes, avocado, tomatoes)
- Vegetables (sweet and white potatoes, dark green leafy vegetables, eggplant, onions)
- Dairy products such as milk and yogurt
- Meats, unsweetened cocoa powder; nuts, dried peas and beans.

Daily recommendations for potassium are 2000 to 5000 mg/day.[242] Some labels list the content, some don't. Strive to eat a few servings daily of the above foods. If you have cardiac or kidney problems, consult your healthcare practitioner regarding potassium intake. A measure of sodium can include:

- 1 teaspoon of salt contains 2300 mg sodium
- 1 teaspoon baking soda contains 1000 mg sodium.[243]

To decrease sodium intake:

- Aim for fresh or frozen fruits and vegetables without added salt.
- Read labels of products for sodium content.
- Have or work towards a meal target of 500 to 700 mg sodium per meal.
- Purchase products with reduced sodium content— many are now the same price as "regular" or "low sodium" foods.
- If you are going to buy snack items, such as pretzels, look for items with no salt added. If that does not appeal to you, mix in half regular, half no salt added. Try something new.
- Give it time. Our bodies take a while to adjust to a lower sodium intake.
- Use fresh or dried herbs, spices, citrus, juices, vinegars, to flavor your foods.
- If you're in the habit of seasoning your food (usually with the salt shaker) before you taste it, replace the salt shaker with a shaker of a different seasoning that has a lower sodium content that straight salt. Try making your own blend with your favorite herbs and spices.
- When dining out, request the salt be left out. Flavor it yourself, and try something new like lemon juice, tobasco, salsa, mustard, vinegar, etc. Of course, if the

sauces/flavorings are loaded with lots of cream, butter, oil, cheese, etc. ask for it on the side, and drizzle rather than pour it on. Chances are a drizzle will give just as much flavor as a pour. Sometimes less, truly is more savoring. Try it!

- For more tips, the *DASH* (Dietary Approaches to Stop Hypertension) *Diet Book*, (Amidon Press) by Marla Heller, MS, RD, offers more tips and plans. You can find it at *www.dashdiet.org*.

Remember this fluid retention note: Many people who get on the scale every day will notice their weight may go up when they didn't eat much. The weight gain could simply be some fluid retention from sodium. Many people consume more than they realize, especially if they eat out often and consume a lot of processed foods.

Recipes

Recipe Acronyms: PRO = Protein; CHO = Carbohydrate; FAT = Fat; Chol = Cholesterol; Gram = gm

Potassium Packed Ratatouille

This recipe is a great accompaniment to meats, poultry, fish, tofu, pasta—any can be mixed in as well. It can also be put in a food processor or blender and used as a dip with crackers, bread, etc.

This recipe tastes even better if made ahead (hours or even a day).

1 small onion, washed and chopped

1 Tbsp olive or canola oil

1 medium eggplant, washed and diced (leaving the skin on is preferable—more antioxidants!)

2 to 3 small-medium zucchini squash, washed and diced

1 package (8-ounces) sliced mushrooms, rinsed

1 can (28-ounces) chopped or crushed tomatoes

1 can (6-ounces) tomato paste

1 tsp. cinnamon

2 tsp. dried or 1-2 Tbsp fresh chopped basil

1/2 tsp. red pepper flakes, optional

2 large clove garlic, peeled and chopped

1/2 cup red wine, optional

In a stockpot, heat oil and onion at medium heat. Cook until tender.

Add eggplant, zucchini, mushrooms, tomatoes and tomato paste.

Add a little water (about 1/2 cup) or wine to prevent scorching. Stir in cinnamon, basil, and red pepper (if desired).

Cover and simmer 20 to 30 minutes or until vegetables are tender. Stir in raw garlic. Makes 6 servings.

Per serving (without wine): 105 Calories, 4 gm PRO, 3 gm FAT, 0 mg Chol, 19 gm CHO, 5 gm Fiber, 540 mg Sodium, 884 mg Potassium.

Metabolic Syndrome

Also known as Syndrome X or Dysmetabolic Syndrome, metabolic syndrome is a cluster of risk factors that are linked to overweight or obesity. It can increase the potential for development of diabetes and heart disease.[244,245]

According to the National Heart Lung and Blood Institute, a person with metabolic syndrome is twice as likely to develop heart disease and five times as likely to develop diabetes as someone without metabolic syndrome.[246] Metabolic syndrome is diagnosed when a person has a combination of at least three of the following risk factors:

- A waistline of 35 inches or more for women and 40 inches or more for men (A large waistline or abdominal obesity—having an apple shape—has been found to put one at greater risk for heart disease—more so than having excess fat in other parts of the body)
- Elevated triglycerides (150 mg/dl or >)
- Low HDL (<50 mg/dl)
- High Blood Pressure (> 130/85 mg/dl)
- Elevated fasting blood glucose (100 mg/dl or >)
- Insulin resistance
- Proinflammatory state (elevated C-reactive protein)
- Increasing age
- Hormone imbalance
- Family history of diabetes
- Gestational diabetes
- Ethnicity/Race-African Americans, Asians, Hispanics and Native Americans tend to have a greater risk.[247-251]

Atherosclerosis (plaque in the arteries and blood vessels) is a condition found with metabolic syndrome. It is thought that elevated insulin levels may promote the plaque buildup. Plaque buildup can lead to clots. Thus, metabolic syndrome does have a link with heart disease.[252-255]

Some cancers have been linked with metabolic syndrome. They include breast, prostate and colon.[256-258]

The incidence of metabolic syndrome is continuing to grow. In the United States alone 25 percent of the population has metabolic syndrome.[259,260] It is preventable.

Treatment of metabolic syndrome includes lifestyle modification, which consist of:

- Regular exercise
- Weight loss
- Stopping smoking
- Following a heart healthy diet, such as a DASH or Mediterranean diet.

Medication may be necessary if lifestyle modification is not effective. This should be discussed with your healthcare practitioner.

Timeout Tip: Just what is a Mediterranean type diet? It is a diet composed of generous amounts of fruits, vegetables, grains, legumes, along with moderate amounts of meats, fish, poultry, dairy products, and wine. Fat intake is primarily from monounsaturated fats, such as olive oil, canola oil, avocado, and nuts. Also, linked with a Mediterranean diet are lifestyle factors. These cultures tend to engage in more physical activity and have a greater social support network. Maybe they just know how to have fun. Remember, laughter is great at lightening things up. One thing you can do anywhere and anytime is smile. It will also relax you.

Recipes

Recipe Acronyms: PRO = Protein; CHO = Carbohydrate; FAT = Fat; Chol = Cholesterol; Gram = gm

Here are a few Mediterranean treats that can be served as a dip with veggies, crackers, or used as a spread on sandwiches or wraps:

Po Boy Pate

1 can (15-ounces) black or kidney beans, washed, rinsed and drained

1 clove garlic, peeled

1 Tbsp. fresh (or 2 tsp. dried) rosemary

1/4 tsp. cumin

1 Tbsp. lemon juice

1 to 2 Tbsp. olive oil

Salt and pepper to taste

In food processor blend all ingredients.

While food processor is on, gradually add olive oil to taste (about 1-2 Tbsp).

Transfer to dish, cover and refrigerate.

Let sit for 20 to 30 minutes for flavors to blend. Salt and pepper to taste if desired. Makes 6 servings.

Per serving: 72 Calories, 3 gm PRO, 9 gm CHO, 3 gm FAT, 0 gm Chol, 3 gm Fiber, 189 mg sodium, 152 mg Potassium.

M.O. Tapenade

1 can (8-ounces) black olives, drained

1 cup sliced fresh mushrooms, rinsed

1/4 cup walnuts

1 red pepper, rinsed, seeded and cut in slices or chunks

1/4 cup fresh parsley

1 Tbsp. lemon juice

1 to 2 Tbsp. olive oil

Salt and pepper to taste

In food processor, blend olives, mushrooms, walnuts, red pepper and parsley. Add lemon juice. Gradually add olive oil to desired texture. Salt and pepper to taste.

Transfer to dish, cover and refrigerate.

Allow flavors to blend for 20 minutes or so. Makes 8 servings.

Per serving: 55 Calories, 1 gm PRO, 3 gm CHO, 5 gm FAT, 0 mg Chol, 1 gm Fiber, 112 mg Sodium, 84 mg Potassium.

Osteoporosis

Osteoporosis is a condition that can cause bones to thin and become weak. *Osteo* means bone and *porosis* means porous, thus porous bone. It is a condition that occurs gradually. In our first few decades of life, bone can break down and be replaced on a regular basis. In our 30s this process begins to slow down. Bones start losing calcium and less "remodeling" takes place. Consequently, bones can become more susceptible to fractures. While osteoporosis can occur at any age, it is more common in those over age 50.[261-263]

The majority of individuals affected by osteoporosis are women. According to the National Institute of Arthritis and Musculoskeletal and Skin Diseases, osteoporosis is a major health threat for over 44 million Americans, 68 percent of which are women.[264] Some experts believe women may have a greater risk of developing osteoporosis due to their bones being lighter and less dense. With menopause, a decrease in estrogen can lead to a decrease in calcium absorption and increased bone resorption.[265-268]

Men are also susceptible. One out of every two women and one out of every four men will have an osteoporosis related fracture in their lifetime.[269]

Risk factors for osteoporosis include:

- Being thin or having a small frame
- Consuming a diet low in calcium
- Physical inactivity
- Overactive thyroid
- Kidney disease
- Cushing's syndrome
- Long term consumption of strong anti-inflammatory drugs used to treat rheumatoid arthritis and asthma
- Women who have their ovaries removed before age 40
- Family history of the disease of fractures after age 50
- Smoking
- Alcohol consumption (2 to 3 ounces per day)[270-273]

Many people with osteoporosis have no idea they have it. Thankfully, we live in a time where it is becoming routine to screen for osteoporosis. A bone mineral density test called a dual-energy x-ray absorptiometry (DXA) measures bone density.[274-277] The test is very similar to having an x-ray.

Many a time individuals are diagnosed with osteopenia. Osteopenia is a condition where the bone density is found to be low. Being diagnosed with osteopenia does not necessarily mean you will develop osteoporosis, however the risk to develop it is greater. Osteopenia can be caused by a few factors including genetics, low bone mass development during adolescence, medical conditions, or treatments that can affect bone health. In the case of either osteopenia or osteoporosis, your healthcare practitioner will likely advise a lifestyle to include regular weight bearing exercise along with a diet to maintain good bone health. Medication may also be prescribed for prevention or treatment of either condition.[278]

Tips to Improve Bone Health

Weight bearing activities can improve bone density. Regular exercise also helps build and maintain muscle mass, along with balance and reaction time. Walking, cycling, jogging, basketball, rollerblading, running, tennis, weight lifting are all examples. Swimming has been shown to have some benefit, although not as much as the weight bearing activities.[279-283]

In some cases individuals are prescribed medications for bone health. These include bisphosphonates, estrogens, calcitonin, and raloxifene and parathyroid hormone.[284]

Nutrition for bone health includes calcium, vitamin D, vitamin K, magnesium, iron, and omega-3 fatty acids; they can all play a role in the absorption of calcium.[285-299]

Calcium is essential for bone health. In 1993, the U.S. Food and Drug Administration (FDA) authorized a health claim related to calcium and osteoporosis for foods and supplements.[300] Ninety nine percent of the body's calcium supply is stored in the bones and teeth where it supports their structure.[301]

Food sources of calcium include dairy products, dark green leafy vegetables (spinach, kale, turnip greens, mustard greens, collard greens), fish with bones, such as sardines, canned salmon (you can mash or puree the bones in a food processor to decrease the risk of choking), tofu fortified with calcium, along with other calcium fortified foods (e.g., calcium fortified orange juice) can contribute to adequate intake. Dairy products are the better absorbed form of calcium.[302]

Another way to increase calcium consumption is the use of vinegar when making soup stock with bones. A little vinegar added to the stock will dissolve some of the calcium from the bones, contributing an added benefit to your soup stock.

When considering calcium supplements, calcium carbonate (for those with normal stomach acid secretion) and calcium citrate (preferably with added vitamin D) are the better absorbed forms. An important point to remember with calcium is that the body can only absorb about 400 to 500 mg of calcium at a time.[303]

Remember that when eating/taking supplements. And consume sources throughout the day.

Daily Calcium Recommendations

According to National Osteoporosis Foundation (NOF) recommendations are:

- Adults under age 50 need 1,000 mg of calcium and 400 to 800 IU of vitamin D daily.
- Adults 50 and over need 1,200 mg of calcium and 800 to 1,000 IU of vitamin D daily.[304]

Vitamin D

In 2010, the FDA expanded the health claim for osteoporosis to include vitamin D. The claim now states, "Adequate calcium and vitamin D as part of a healthful diet, along with physical activity, may reduce the risk of osteoporosis in later life."[305]

Vitamin D in particular plays a large role in the absorption of calcium. Many foods have it added. Sources include vitamin D fortified dairy and cereal products, egg yolks, and fish such as salmon, sardines, catfish, and tuna. Another source of it is sunshine. Those who live in sunnier climates tend to have a better chance of absorbing the light that creates this vitamin, thus improving calcium absorption. Many who live in the northern climates have less exposure to sunlight, particularly in winter. Fifteen minutes of sun a few days per week (before applying sunscreen) can help the body produce vitamin D. Read more information in "The Importance of Vitamin D" section in Chapter 3 of this book.

Vitamin K

Vitamin K comes in two forms, K1 and K2. K1 is the form which is involved in normal blood clotting. K2 is the more potent of the two and plays a role in maintaining bone metabolism. Another role K2 plays is in circulatory health. It assists in protecting arteries from calcification (plaque build-up). Sources of K1 include green leafy vegetables and plant oils, such as soybean and canola. K2 can be found in fermented soybeans (natto), dairy products, and egg yolks. The dietary reference intake (DRI) for vitamin K is 120 IU for men and 90 IU for women over 30.[306-308]

An important note for those taking anti-clotting agents, such as Coumadin/Warfarin: a high intake of vitamin K is not recommended as it can interfere with this medication. Discuss this with your health-care practitioner.

Magnesium

Magnesium has been linked to improving bone mineral density and quality. According to the National Institute of Arthritis and Musculoskeletal and Skin Diseases, "60 percent of the magnesium in our bodies is found in our bones in combination with calcium and phosphorus."[309] Magnesium has been linked to blood pressure reduction, and a low intake of magnesium may also be linked to Type 2 Diabetes. The DRI for magnesium is 420 mg/day for males over 30, and 320 mg/day for females over 30. Sources include green leafy vegetables, nuts, seeds, whole grains and chocolate. Some antacids and laxatives also contain magnesium. While it is safe to consume high levels of magnesium in food, excessive supplementation (>350 mg/day) may be toxic.[310,311]

Phosphorus

Phosphorus is another mineral that plays a key role in not only bone health but tissue growth. Eighty-five percent of phosphorus is found in our bones. The DRI is 700 mg for men and women over 30. Dairy products, meat, eggs, poultry, cola beverages, and many processed foods contain phosphorus. If calcium intake is low and phosphorus intake is high, it may interfere with calcium absorption. The *Tolerable Upper Intake* is 4000 mg/day for individuals 9 to 70 years of age; after age 70 it is 3000 mg/day.[312]

Iron

Iron plays a role in the strength of our bones by assisting certain enzymes in the formation of the bone matrix. The DRI for iron is 8 mg for men over age 19; it is 18 mg for women age 19 to 50, and 8 mg for women over 50. Intake over 45 mg/day is not recommended. The heme form of iron is the better absorbed and is found in red meat, shellfish, liver, and poultry. Non-heme sources of iron include canned beans, green leafy vegetables, and fortified foods. Calcium can interfere with iron absorption; vitamin C, however, can enhance it. If you are taking supplements of either kind, taking calcium and iron at a separate time of day will assist in the improved absorption of each mineral.[313] Keep in mind iron supplements can cause gastric upset or constipation.

Here are a couple of mealtime examples to assist in optimum absorption:

- **A cheese and spinach omelet:** Eggs contain iron. Spinach contains some calcium and iron. Cheese contains calcium. To improve the iron absorption of the eggs and spinach, accompany the omelet with a glass of citrus fruit or juice, tomato juice, strawberries or kiwifruit.
- **Having a cheeseburger:** Beef contains iron. Cheese contains calcium. Accompany the burger with some broccoli or cabbage slaw and red or green peppers. A few extra slices of tomato can boost vitamin C content as well. A refreshing dessert of mixed berries and melon also provide a boost of vitamin C. (Of course, vitamin C is available in supplement form. The DRI is 75 mg/day for women and 90 mg/day for men. The food source seems like a lot more fun though.)

To be sure, there are additional compounds that contribute to our bone health than those listed above. Some of these include boron, copper, fluoride, isoflavones, and zinc. In the meantime, eating a variety of foods can make a difference in our health and keep us standing strong!

> For more information regarding bone health, you can refer to the National Institutes for Health Osteoporosis and Related Bone Diseases. The website is *www.niams.nih.gov/Health_Info/bone/default.asp*. Other websites are: National Osteoporosis Foundation, *www.nof.org*, and the National Institute of Arthritis and Musculoskeletal and Skin Disease, *www.osteo.org*.

Snack Ideas

- How about a glass of ice cold milk (or homemade chocolate milk with unsweetened cocoa powder and add sweetener to taste)?
- Calcium fortified orange juice along with a few crackers and a slice of cheese
- Cup of plain yogurt with cereal and nuts
- String cheese with an apple, pear, or grapes
- Melted Brie cheese with sliced apple or pear on toast

Recipes

Recipe Acronyms: PRO = Protein; CHO = Carbohydrate; FAT = Fat; Chol = Cholesterol; Gram = gm

Broccoli and Carrot Bisque

2 cloves garlic, peeled and chopped

1 Tbsp. fresh grated ginger (or 2 tsp. dried)

2 Tbsp. olive, canola or Enova oil

1 small onion, washed, peeled and chopped

1/4 tsp. black pepper

1 tsp. turmeric

2 tsp. dried oregano

1 tsp curry powder, optional

1 lb. broccoli florets washed, and broken into small pieces

1 lb. carrots, washed, peeled and cut into 1/2-inch slices

2 cups stock or broth (can be chicken or vegetable) or instant made with 2 tsp. instant bouillon (or 1 bouillon cube)

2 cups lowfat milk

2 Tbsp. flour

Options for garnish: Sour cream, plain yogurt, grated cheese, snipped chives

In a stockpot, place oil, garlic, spices and oregano.

Heat until slightly cooked over medium heat. Add broccoli, carrots, and stock/broth.

Cover and cook over medium heat until vegetables are tender, but not overcooked.

Remove from heat.

Spoon batches of vegetables (about 2 cups at a time) in a blender or food processor until blended, but not runny.

Place into a large bowl until all vegetables are pureed.

In a small bowl, mix milk into flour gradually until flour is dissolved.

Return stockpot to stove and medium high heat.

Add milk mixture to stockpot, and allow liquids to thicken, but not boil.

Add vegetable mixture to milk mixture in stockpot and mix all ingredients. Serve hot.

Garnish with a dollop of sour cream or yogurt and some freshly snipped chives, or a sprinkle (about 1 Tbsp.) grated cheese.

A great accompaniment would be to serve with some hearty whole-grain bread or rolls along with some olive oil, balsamic vinegar and dried oregano for dipping bread. Makes 6 servings.

Per serving: 155 Calories, 7 gm PRO, 19 gm CHO, 7 gm FAT, 7 mg Chol, 4 gm Fiber, 168 mg Calcium, 325 mg Sodium, 680 mg Potassium.

Hormonal Changes, Appetite and Moods

One of the more, shall we say, "interesting" changes we boomers are starting to experience is minor lapses in our memory. Research indicates that for many of us these "moments or lapses" occur due to a decreased level of hormones. Hormones have a number of functions. A few of them include our appetites, moods, mental clarity and energy levels.[314-316]

A few hormones involved in appetite regulation include leptin, ghrelin, dopamine, and cortisol. Leptin is a hormone that signals satisfaction to our brain and tells us we are full. It is also known as the satiety hormone.[317,318] Dopamine is a neurotransmitter.[319] It plays a role in motivation, addiction, and reward (it makes us feel good).[320] While dopamine is released at the first bite of food and signals us to eat more, leptin quiets that impulse.[321-323] Ghrelin is a hormone secreted in the stomach. It signals the cells in the brain's appetite center that we are hungry.[324] It has been found that people who don't get enough sleep have elevated levels of ghrelin (making us hungry) and lower levels of leptin (which turns hunger signals off).[325,326] Many people who experience insomnia tend to gain weight due to these sneaky processes going on. Now we know why. Food gives us energy and can wake us up. With elevated levels of ghrelin circulating in our bodies along with being groggy from lack of sleep, it's no wonder we turn to food.

Another hormone is cortisol. Cortisol is a stress hormone, and is produced by the adrenal glands.[327,328] Levels in our bodies fluctuate throughout the day and when they are low that may stimulate hunger. Many of us experience an afternoon lull of energy, and it could be due to a decrease in cortisol, as it typically drops at this point in the day. If you can get up and move around, and/or have a snack with balance (protein, carbohydrate, fat, and fiber—a half sandwich, cheese or nut butter and crackers, a cup of sugar-free yogurt), this may help stave off any craving induced by the energy lull. As many of us already know, it takes about 20 minutes for the brain to receive signal that we have eaten and our ghrelin levels will (finally) fall. Eating slower can help alleviate some of the overeating urge many of us experience, but it can be difficult when we are famished, stressed, or in a hurry.

A way to keep some of the mood and energy swings under control is to be mindful of what you eat. Christiane Northrup, MD, author of *The Wisdom of Menopause* and *Women's Bodies Women's Wisdom*, (Random House), suggests reducing sodium, sugar, and white flour. For some, cutting back on caffeine may also help alleviate some of the ups and downs that are already going on in our bodies.[329] Women are not alone in hormonal changes. Men experience a decrease in testosterone in their late 40s and early 50s.

While there is no defined set of symptoms for male menopause (*sometimes referred to as andropause*) some do experience symptoms similar to women.[330,331] A few lifestyle changes may help alleviate some of the symptoms that coincide with "the change." In the "Got the Blues and No Rhythm" section in this chapter, a few more tips on beating the blues are reviewed. While our energy levels may wax and wane, endorphins can still be produced, and they make us feel good. Exercise, laughter, and sex can release them.

Another thing hormonal fluctuations can do is impair our sleep. In females, the hormone progesterone plays a role in inducing sleep. Some women may notice they sleep better during the second half of their menstrual cycle, as progesterone levels are higher. During menopause, the fluctuation in hormone levels, along with hot flashes can also impair sleep.[332]

Getting through this phase of life is like a long train ride. There is a light at the end of the tunnel, however. Mood swings subside, hot flashes go away, sleep may improve, and you may feel human again!

As we all have our own set of circumstances, it is important to discuss options with your healthcare practitioner.

Sleep Disorders

Sleep deprivation can not only cause fatigue, but can also affect daily activities, motor skills, memory, and mood. Just like food, air and water, we need adequate sleep every day.

There are two types of sleep: Rapid Eye Movement (REM) and non-REM. They each have their purpose. And, in the course of sleep, our bodies go through a series of distinct stages and predictable patterns, all of which are necessary for a good night's rest.

Surprisingly, the need for sleep is not just for rest. During sleep, our body actually becomes quite active, and a number of functions take place. The brain is very active throughout sleep.[333,334]

One process that occurs is certain hormones are released which heighten pathways in the brain to enhance learning and memory. Another process that occurs is the production of cytokines, which are hormones that help boost our immune function. Many people who do not get enough sleep have an impaired ability to fight infections.[335,336]

Throughout the course of the sleep cycle, overall our heart rate and blood pressure are reduced by about 10 percent. If we do not regularly get enough sleep there may be an increased risk for stroke, angina, irregular heartbeat and heart attacks.[337-339] A lack of sleep may also increase the release of cortisol, adrenaline and other stress hormones, which may contribute to an increased risk for heart disease by not allowing for blood pressure reduction during sleep cycles. Some research has shown that individuals who chronically do not get enough sleep have higher levels of C-reactive protein.[340] As mentioned in the Cardiovascular Disease section, C-reactive protein has been linked with an increase risk of developing atherosclerosis. There has also been an association of an increase in obesity, depression and diabetes due to lack of sleep and overeating.[341,342]

According to the American Sleep Association about 60 million Americans have insomnia frequently or for extended periods of time; 40 million suffer from chronic long-term sleep disorders each year.[343] While many feel insomnia may be due to stress or worry, this may not always be the case. Insomnia may be due to a physical problem. According to a nationwide study by the Association of Sleep Disorders Centers, physical ailments—such as disorders of breathing or abnormal muscle activity—are often the cause of sleep disruption and may account for a large number of self-diagnosed cases of insomnia.

As we age, we tend to spend less time in the deep restful stages of sleep. Additionally the quality of our sleep may be reduced due to health conditions such as arthritis, heart conditions, anxiety, depression, stress, GERD, and medications.[344,345] Something as simple as waking up in the middle of the night to urinate can cause a disturbance in sleep. Many of us know all too well the effects of not having a good night's rest. Your healthcare practitioner may suggest keeping a sleep diary and review it with you to assist in finding the possible cause of insomnia. There are lots of remedies out there to help improve our sleep. These include:

- Eating the majority of your protein intake early in the day. Protein has amino acids that help keep us awake throughout the day.
- Consuming a meal with carbohydrates a few hours prior to going to sleep. Carbohydrates allow for the release of serotonin, which can make us sleepy (see Carbohydrate section in Chapter 6). Try to eat something that will not be too heavy or a stimulant, such as a spicy or sugary food. A few snack ideas include a bowl of cereal or oatmeal, fruit with milk, nuts, cheese, or unsweetened yogurt, half sandwich, cheese and crackers.
- Eating two to four hours prior to bedtime, and avoiding large meals prior to bedtime.
- Limiting caffeine and alcohol consumption. Try eliminating the caffeine after lunch or by mid-afternoon—its effect can last for 8 to 10 hours, depending on your sensitivity. Alcohol may induce sleep, but the after effect can cause a rebound and wake you up; you may also have a less restful sleep.
- Exercising in the morning or at least five or six hours prior to bedtime.
- Try to establish a consistent time of day to go to sleep. The body does adapt better to a consistent sleep schedule.
- If you do wake up and cannot fall asleep, it is recommended to go into another room and do something that can help relax you before going back to bed.
- Turning off and unplugging the television or any other electrical device such as a computer, DVD, VCR, as they may disturb your ability to fall and stay asleep. Also try to keep cell phones or telephones as far away from your bed as possible.
- We live in a time where our environment has a great deal of electricity and electromagnetic radiation (EMR)

emitted from devices, such as computers, cell phones, etc. When an appliance is turned off but plugged in there is still an electrical current running through the wires. While more research needs to be confirmed as the effect this has on our bodies, powering down when you go to sleep is worth experimenting with.

- Evidence shows that light can cause our bodies to wake up. It's all about our circadian rhythm and light signaling us to be awake. Sleep in a dark room. Try using eye covers to block out any extra light, or install light blocking draperies/blinds. Turn the electric alarm clock away from you, as the light can interfere with your sleep.
- Some herbal teas, such as chamomile, or some warm milk can help us relax and fall asleep.
- Ask your healthcare practitioner about valerian, melatonin or 5-hydroxytryptophan (5-HTP). For some, these products may help induce sleep.
- Relaxation exercises can help us unwind and clear our thoughts.
- Naps may help, but not after 3 pm. Taking naps after 3 pm may impair your ability to fall asleep.
- Keep the temperature of the room a little on the cooler side.
- If you're waking up with a stiff or achy back, maybe you need to flip your mattress (or get a new one).
- Change your pillows every six months to a year.
- Try some lavender. Whether a mist, aromatherapy, lotion or some sprigs by the bedside.[346-348]
- In some cases your healthcare practitioner will prescribe medication to help you sleep.

Sleep Apnea

Another fairly common sleep disorder is sleep apnea. Sleep apnea is a condition where there are pauses in breathing during sleep.

There are two types of sleep apnea. The first and more common is *Obstructive Sleep Apnea* (OSA), which occurs when the soft tissue at the back of the throat collapses during sleep, thus blocking the airway.[349-351] Due to the lack of oxygen, your brain wakes you up. When normal breathing starts again, many times it is with a choking or snoring type sound. While many people who snore do have sleep apnea, it is not always the case. The second is *Central Sleep Apnea,* which is due to some type of instability in the respiratory center and the brain fails to signal the muscles to breathe.[352-354]

Due to intermittent oxygen level reduction and reduced quality of sleep, there is an increase in stress hormones. And, as mentioned earlier, this can lead to an increased risk of high blood pressure, risk of stroke, heart attacks, and congestive heart failure. Additionally the reduction of oxygen can lead to morning headaches, an impaired ability to concentrate, think clearly, learn, and remember. Mood disorders and depression can also occur. The risk of an automobile or work related accident is tripled due to lack of restful sleep.[355-357]

It is estimated that between 12 and 18 million Americans adults suffer from sleep apnea. Over half the people who experience it are overweight. And it is more common in men. While sleep apnea can occur at any age, one in 25 middle age men and one in 50 women have it. It occurs more often with Hispanics, African Americans, Asians, and Native Americans than with Caucasians.[358,359] Other factors in sleep apnea include:

- Family history of sleep apnea
- Congestion due to allergies that can narrow airways
- Enlarged tonsils and adenoids
- Throat muscles and tongue that relax more than normal while asleep

- Head and neck shape that creates a smaller airway size in the mouth and throat area

Many people with sleep apnea have no idea they have it. They tend to feel tired throughout the day. To be diagnosed for sleep apnea, it is necessary to be monitored, usually through a sleep center. There are treatment strategies for sleep apnea. They include:

- If overweight, reduce body weight.
- Sleep on your side versus your back.
- Avoid alcohol, smoking, sleeping pills, herbal supplements, or any other medication that makes you sleepy. These substances may make it more difficult for your airway to stay open while you sleep.
- With moderate or severe sleep apnea, Continuous Positive Airway Pressure (CPAP) is utilized. CPAP is a mask worn while sleeping that is hooked up to a machine that delivers air continuously. It allows for a constant airflow into the nostrils. CPAP provides for continuous airway pressure to allow the airways in the nostril and mouth to stay open. If discontinued, sleep apnea will likely return.[360-362]

For more information go to the American Sleep Association at *www.sleepassociation.org*.

Got the Blues and No Rhythm?

To say we live in a world with a little stress is an understatement. In a January 2006 telephone survey conducted by the American Psychological Association, 50 percent of working Americans revealed that they are concerned about their level of stress.

Stress has been linked to many ailments, including hypertension, obesity, depression, headaches, sleep disturbances, gastrointestinal ailments, and the list goes on.[363] We experience it at home and at work. Some of us can cope with it better than others. Of course, some days are better than others, as we all know. As previously mentioned, exercise can help relieve stress and its effects. It can help release neurochemicals in the body known as endorphins to help relax the body and mind.[364-366] How many of us can relate to the fact that when we are stressed and we literally walk away from the situation for a little while it can look better? Going to the gym, socializing with friends, yoga, meditation, lifting weights, getting a massage, a hobby, whatever—it is good for the body and the soul. We all need down time to just relax and recharge.

Another factor that can help elevate our moods is sunshine, particularly in winter. Many people experience seasonal affective disorder (SAD). With less daylight, and colder temperatures, that can bring on the blues. Getting 15 to 20 minutes daily of sunshine has been shown to be effective in elevating our moods. While there are many climates that don't have much sunshine in winter months, special lights designed to mimic sunlight can provide some relief. Vitamin D supplements can provide the nutrition boost many may need who cannot obtain enough sunlight.[367] As mentioned in the vitamin D section, Chapter 3, there may be a link between mood and vitamin D.

Another set of compounds that have been linked with mood is omega-3 fatty acids. Some evidence shows that consuming omega-3 fatty acids may boost those blues.[368] Another study revealed that a high intake of omega-6 fatty acids showed a link with heart disease and depression. Omega-6 fatty acids are found in processed foods and refined oils. Omega-6 intake has increased markedly over the last century. The ratio of omega-6 to omega-3 in hunter-gatherer times was *two* to *three* omega-6: one omega-3. Now, however it is thought to be 15 to 17 times more omega-6 to omega-3. The study was published in *Psychosomatic Medicine*.[369]

Additional factors that can play a role in our mindset include environmental toxins, such as petrochemicals, heavy metals, molds, allergens, diet, digestive disturbances, hormonal fluctuations and infections. Any one of these can create an imbalance in our body chemistry, thus affecting our behavior. It is important to find a healthcare practitioner who knows how to help you learn what may be going on in your body. A simple adjustment of diet, nutritional supplements, and in some cases, medication, may help offset the imbalance you may be experiencing.

You owe it to yourself to be good to your body and mind. Where was it ever written we are supposed to walk around all stressed out and blue? Be selfish for yourself. For many of us, we may feel that our health ailments are inherited, and there is no way to treat them. Au contraire! Help and treatment is now available, and science is sure to continue to improve ways to detect and treat factors to improve our health and well being.

Skin Care

Skin is our largest organ. It helps regulate body temperature and provides us with protection from the elements and some infections.[370]

One of the first places aging starts to show up is the skin. As we age, our skin loses its elasticity. Hormonal changes, exposure to sunlight, stress, and lifestyle factors also play a role.[371-376]

Here are a few tips to help maintain the health and glow of your skin:

- **Stop smoking.** Smoking reduces blood flow and can interfere with wound healing.[377]
- **Use a good sunscreen.** Some of the damage showing up on our skin in our forties and beyond may be due to sun

exposure from our childhood. Effects can include wrinkling, blotchy pigmentation and skin cancer. A sunscreen with an SPF of at least 15 applied every few hours when outside is what dermatologists recommend. Ultraviolet radiation (UV) comes in two forms: UVA and UVB. Agents that protect against both UVA and UVB rays include zinc oxide and titanium dioxide. Some sunscreens also contain antioxidants, such as vitamin C, E, or green tea that may help to improve the texture and tone of the skin. [378-380] For more information on recommended sunscreens refer to the Skin Cancer Foundation at *www.skincancer.org.*

- **Reduce your intake of sugar and simple carbs.** Evidence reveals that sugar consumption may play a role in the development of wrinkles. Leslie Baumann, MD, author of *The Skin Type Solution*, states that "Sugar triggers a natural process called glycation, which is the same chemical reaction that turns meat brown when you cook it. The sugars bind with tissues to form harmful molecules, called advanced glycation end products (AGE's), which damage elastin and collagen—two substances skin needs to stay supple and elastic."[381] Sugar may also play a role in interfering with antioxidant-protecting enzymes that help protect skin from sun damage.[382]

  The effects of sugar on the skin start to show around age thirty-five and appear to become more apparent over time, according to a 2007 study in the *British Journal of Dermatology*. Foods with a high glycemic index, such as white potatoes, pasta, along with candy and sugary foods and beverages contribute to the process.[383]

- **Exercise and manage stress.** Exercise increases circulation and can also reduce stress. Both circulation and stress reduction can be of benefit to the skin. Stress can lead to increased production of epinephrine, which can cause a constriction of blood vessels, causing skin to lose its glow, according to Naila Malik, MD, a cosmetic dermatologist.[384]

- **Eat well.** Consume foods rich in vitamin C, which, according to Toby Amidor, RD, director of nutrition for DietTV.com in New York City, helps support the structure of skin through production of collagen. Sources of vitamin C include: citrus, kiwi fruit, berries, cantaloupe, mango, papaya, tomatoes, dark green leafy vegetables, peppers, broccoli, and cabbage. Vitamin E is another antioxidant that may promote skin protection. Sources of vitamin E are: sunflower seeds, almonds, hazelnuts, peanut butter, wheat germ, and dark green leafy vegetables. Beta carotene, which converts to vitamin A, also helps promote healthy skin. Sources of vitamin A are: carrots, sweet potatoes, pumpkin, cantaloupe, broccoli, pink grapefruit, apricots, and dark green leafy vegetables.

  - **Stay hydrated.** Consume adequate amounts of liquid so you are not thirsty. Many fruits and vegetables contain fluid, plus juices, beverages, soups, and water. Some experts suggest consuming at least 6 eight-ounce glasses of water per day in addition to other sources mentioned. **Note:** Excessive amounts of alcohol can cause dehydration.

  - **Consume adequate protein.** Protein is a building block of skin. Many protein sources also include iron and zinc, both of which are a part of cell growth and contribute to skin health. Good sources of protein are: beef, beans, eggs, oysters, dark meat of chicken, salmon, and tuna.

- ○ **The flavonols in cocoa** have been shown to help improve circulation, and also reduce blood pressure. So, consuming a cup of homemade cocoa (see recipe on page 97) or some chocolate with at least 70% cacao might be something to consider.[385-391]
- **Moisturize.** There are a number of moisturizers available that help promote skin health. Some contain retinoids (which are derivatives of vitamin A, e.g., Retin-A®), alpha-hydroxy-acids, cosmeceuticals that contain antioxidants (such as vitamin C), peptides, and botanicals.
- **Get adequate rest.** According to dermatologist Nicholas Perricone, MD, getting enough sleep helps with the production of human growth hormone (HGH), which helps keep skin more elastic. Also sleeping on your back can reduce sleep lines that are formed when sleeping on your side.[392]
- **Perform regular skin exams.** If you think something has changed on your skin, have it checked. Your healthcare practitioner may also perform a skin exam along with your annual physical.

Or, to find a dermatologist in your area go to the American Academy of Dermatology at *http://www.aad.org/*.

Be Well Boomer!

Appendix A

Adult BMI Chart

Locate the height of interest in the left-most column and read across the row for that height to the weight of interest. Follow the column of the weight up to the top row that lists the BMI. BMI of 18.5-24.9 is the healthy weight range, BMI of 25-29.9 is the overweight range, and BMI of 30 and above is in the obese range.

Adult BMI Chart

BMI	19	20	21	22	23	24	25	26	27	28	29	30	31	32	33	34	35
Height									Weight in Pounds								
4'10"	91	96	100	105	110	115	119	124	129	134	138	143	148	153	158	162	167
4'11"	94	99	104	109	114	119	124	128	133	138	143	148	153	158	163	168	173
5'	97	102	107	112	118	123	128	133	138	143	148	153	158	163	158	174	179
5'1"	100	106	111	116	122	127	132	137	143	148	153	158	164	169	174	180	185
5'2"	104	109	115	120	126	131	136	142	147	153	158	164	169	175	180	186	191
5'3"	107	113	118	124	130	135	141	146	152	158	163	169	175	180	186	191	197
5'4"	110	116	122	128	134	140	145	151	157	163	169	174	180	186	192	197	204
5'5"	114	120	126	132	138	144	150	156	162	168	174	180	186	192	198	204	210
5'6"	118	124	130	136	142	148	155	161	167	173	179	186	192	198	204	210	216
5'7"	121	127	134	140	146	153	159	166	172	178	185	191	198	204	211	217	223
5'8"	125	131	138	144	151	158	164	171	177	184	190	197	203	210	216	223	230
5'9"	128	135	142	149	155	162	169	176	182	189	196	203	209	216	223	230	236
5'10"	132	139	146	153	160	167	174	181	188	195	202	209	216	222	229	236	243
5'11"	136	143	150	157	165	172	179	186	193	200	208	215	222	229	236	243	250
6'	140	147	154	162	169	177	184	191	199	206	213	221	228	235	242	250	258
6'1"	144	151	159	166	174	182	189	197	204	212	219	227	235	242	250	257	265
6'2"	148	155	163	171	179	186	194	202	210	218	225	233	241	249	256	264	272
6'3"	152	160	168	176	184	192	200	208	216	224	232	240	248	256	264	272	279
	Healthy Weight						Overweight					Obese					

Source: Evidence Report of Clinical Guidelines on the Identification, Evaluation, and Treatment of Overweight and Obesity in Adults, 1998. NIH/National Heart, Lung, and Blood Institute (NHLBI).

http:www.health.gov/DietaryGuidelines/dga2005/document/html/chapter3.htm

Appendix B

Foods that Pack a Nutritional Punch

Here is a list of food items that pack a nutritional punch. Incorporate as many of them as possible into your daily diet:

Acai—Found primarily in the Amazon River communities, acai packs a plethora of nutrition. These include antioxidants such an anthocyanins, omega-9 fatty acids, and phytosterols; and minerals such as calcium and iron; vitamin A; and fiber.

Apples—Contain the antioxidants quercetin and pectin, a great source of fiber. Dark-red-skinned red apples contain higher amounts of antioxidants. Remember the skins of most fruits and vegetables have the color, which contains more antioxidants. So, wash them well and chow down!

Avocadoes—A great source of monounsaturated fat. Avocado can be used as a dip or spread, and served in a salad. It is a great alternative to mayonnaise. Lemon and lime juice really pop the flavor of avocado.

Blueberries—Loaded with heart-healthy soluble fiber, blueberries have been found to promote memory retention as they contain flavonoids. Fresh, frozen, or canned, blueberries can stand out on their own and make a great snack or dish. They can also be used as a topping, added to cereals, used in smoothies, pies, etc.

Beans (Black, Garbanzo, Kidney, Pinto, etc.)—Great source of protein, heart-healthy soluble fiber, and minerals. The darker-skinned beans contain more antioxidants. Black, kidney, and pinto beans contain more iron. The sky is the limit with beans, as you can use them in soups, salads, burritos, spreads.

Capsaicin—An ingredient found in hot peppers, capsaicin is thought to increase metabolic rate slightly and has been shown to potentially help reduce growth of the prostate cancer cell. Also something to remember when you have a cold— spicy food can cause a runny nose thus relieving congestion. Add a few drops of hot sauce or hot pepper to perk up soup or most any other dish. Fruit salads, salsa, soups, starch dishes, casseroles, meats, etc. are all more exciting when they have some heat. Another perk is the heat from spicy dishes tends to make you feel fuller sooner.

Cherries—Rich in taste and anthocyanins, an antioxidant that may play a role in revving up your immune system, cherries may reduce inflammation associated with arthritis and gout. Eat them fresh, canned, or dried. Add them to cereal, salads, baked goods, etc.

Chocolate—A heavenly creation that makes the world a better place. Dark chocolate has the antioxidant benefits (look for at least 60 to 70 percent cocoa content in a chocolate bar). See *Cocoa.*

Chromium—Chromium is a mineral thought to be a great help in controlling blood glucose levels, especially for diabetics. Good sources of chromium are egg yolks, bran, yeast, black pepper, whole grains, broccoli, and meat.

Cinnamon—A spice that helps control blood glucose (sugar) and cholesterol levels, also helps with blood pressure control. Additional studies show cinnamon can improve cognitive function; simply smelling the spice alerted the brain and helped reduce fatigue, along with improving memory, coordination, and attention.

Citrus—In addition to a great source of vitamin C, citrus provides folate, potassium, soluble, heart-healthy fiber, and other antioxidants (flavonoids, carotenoids) that can help inhibit tumor growth and protect vision health. Wash citrus before peeling, slicing, or grating, and enjoy these fruits in everything from water to sauces, salads, and baked goods.

Cocoa—This compound has wonderful heart-health attributes, such as lowering blood pressure, and on a simplistic level, creates a sense of calm in people. In ancient cultures, cocoa was used to quell diarrhea and other digestive disorders. Cocoa has antioxidants (flavonoids) that can help relax blood vessels. The most common use of cocoa is in producing chocolate. It can also be used in rubs/seasonings and makes great sauces, such as mole. Another common use for cocoa is in hot chocolate and chocolate milk.

Coffee—Coffee contains as many if not more antioxidants than blueberries or broccoli. Additionally, studies show that drinking a few cups of coffee (ground, without added milk, sugar, etc.; not Scandinavian style, which is boiling beans, or the French press method) a day has been linked with decreasing cavities, elevating mood, improving headaches, helping to increase endurance and decrease fatigue. Lastly coffee has been linked with a reduction in liver cancer, cirrhosis of the liver, colon cancer, gallstones, Parkinson's disease—and in larger amounts (six cups per day), it has been shown to reduce the risk of type 2 diabetes. On the flipside, drinking a lot of coffee has been shown to cause jitters in people sensitive to caffeine; people prone to osteoporosis or sleep disturbances may want to discuss coffee intake with their healthcare practitioner. Bottom line, for most people a few cups of java a day is okay.

Cranberries—Cranberries have been shown to help prevent bacteria from sticking in the bladder. They can be added to everything from cereals, snacks, baked goods, and used as a garnish.

EGCG—Epigallocatechin gallate is a flavonoid, and one of the potent compounds found in green and black tea. These compounds have the property of reducing inflammation, as well as improving blood flow. Green tea contains 30 to 40 percent; black tea contains 3 to10 percent. Adding milk to tea can potentially neutralize the antioxidant benefits, so keep that in mind.

Flax—Source of omega-3 fatty acids and a good source of fiber. Flaxseed has been shown to help lower the risk of heart disease and arrhythmias along with boosting immunity. Buying flaxseed and grinding it (the whole seed is difficult to digest) at home is the best way to ensure a fresh product.

Add ground flaxseed to cereals, baked goods, salads, smoothies, casseroles, and meat loaf; mix with nuts, dried fruit, and dark chocolate chunks to top on plain yogurt or ice cream. The sky is the limit!

Garlic—Provides possible cardiovascular benefits, and has been shown to decrease plaque formation in the arteries and anti-infective properties. The benefit is in the raw product thus you should add some raw garlic at the end of cooking to benefit from its properties.

Ginger—The active compound in ginger is gingerol, which has been shown to assist in conditions ranging from nausea and motion sickness to heart disease, certain cancers, arthritis, and Alzheimer's disease. Fresh ginger has much more flavor than powdered, but both are great. Ginger can be used on meats; fish; poultry; vegetables; soups; beverages; sauces; rice; pasta; and desserts, such as cookies, fruit and nut breads, and cakes.

Grains—Whole grains are loaded with satisfaction. Not only do you feel satiated and satisfied when you eat them, they contain soluble and insoluble fiber, which is great in aiding your heart, digestive system, and providing quick and sustained energy.

Greens—Spinach, collards, kale, turnip, and mustard are great sources of nutrient density, including vitamin A and lutein (good for the eyes). Some added fat, such as olive oil, can boost absorption. Tossing greens into salads adds color and nutrition.

Mushrooms—A high-nutrient density and low-calorie food. Mushrooms contain B vitamins, selenium, potassium, and copper. They are loaded with heart-healthy antioxidant compounds.

Nuts—A satisfying snack food and a great source of omega-3 fats and protein. Shown to be heart-healthy and sustain energy, nuts can be added to just about anything—salads, cereal, snack mixes, desserts, and stir-fry dishes, etc.

Oats—Source of soluble fiber, oats are associated with lowering the LDL (low density lipoproteins) cholesterol. Sprinkle oats with cinnamon, flaxseed, walnuts, and dried fruit (cherries, cranberries, raisins, blueberries, apricots) and you have a meal loaded with antioxidants and fiber. Use oats in conjunction with flour when baking. For example, in a cookie recipe, use half oatmeal/ground oatmeal and half flour. Your body will be ever so grateful!

Oils—Remember, you need fat for good health. Heart healthier oils are those high in omega-3 fatty acids. The trick is they break down and oxidize faster than their omega-6 counterparts. Omega-3 oils include canola, walnut, flaxseed (flaxseed oil is best utilized when not cooked, as it has a low smoking point—salads are a great use for flaxseed oil). Olive oil is a fantastic oil. Loaded with anti-inflammatory properties and monounsaturated fat, olive oil is delicious in salads. It has a lower smoking point, so use olive oil when sautéing. Enova oil is relatively new to the U.S. A blend of soybean and canola oils, it has been used in Japan for quite some time. In a nutshell, Enova oil is less absorbed as a fat than regular fats. It has a high smoking point as well (420°F). Canola oil also has a higher smoking point, so can be used in broiling, grilling, etc.

Oregano—On a comparative gram-per-gram basis, fresh oregano has 42 times more antioxidant activity than an apple, 12 times more than an orange, and 4 times more than blueberries. Use oregano in rice, pasta, casseroles, salads, meat dishes, fish, etc.

Pomegranates—Loaded with antioxidants, pomegranates contain polyphenols and anthocyanins. Polyphenols are potent antioxidants that may possess heart-protective and anti-cancer (particularly the prostate) properties. Anthocyanins also possess anti-inflammatory benefits. The fresh fruit can be eaten as is or added to salads, rice, or couscous dishes, fruit salads, ice cream, yogurt, and cereal. Pomegranate juice can be used as is or mixed with other fruit juices. Some folks enjoy pomegranate martinis.

Raspberries—A powerhouse of antioxidants. In a study published in the journal *BioFactors,* the antioxidant compounds hold up even under processing and storage. Raspberries add flavor, color, and fiber to any dish. Add them to cereal, salads, baked goods, yogurt, ice cream, etc.

225

Rosemary—This herb contains antioxidants and phenolic compounds which may promote circulation and brain stimulation. Rosemary adds wonderful flavor to meats, stews, starches, and dips.

Seafood—Fatty fish such as salmon, mackerel, tuna, and sardines have the potent omega-3 fatty acids that help reduce inflammation. Fish has also been shown to possibly benefit the brain and the condition of ADHD. It is recommended to strive for two to three servings per week of fish. Some fish, however, contain environmental contaminants, such as mercury. Fish with the highest levels of mercury are those that are larger, such as shark, swordfish, tilefish, and king mackerel.

Sweet Potatoes—A source of carotene and fiber. How about a baked sweet potato with a drizzle of olive oil or a teaspoon of butter and some cinnamon sprinkled on top? Yum—sort of like having your vegetable and dessert together!

Tomatoes—A source of lycopene, which has been shown to possibly help prevent prostate cancer, along with other cancers, and heart disease. It is better absorbed when the tomatoes are cooked.

Turmeric—This spice is quickly becoming of interest in the effects it may have on many conditions ranging from arthritis, heart disease, cancer, and Alzheimer's. The compound piperine, found in black pepper, enhances absorption of the antioxidants in turmeric. While there are many applications for use of this spice, I suggest adding it to egg salad, grain dishes, veggies, and in dressings.

Vinegar—Shown to help in blood sugar control, vinegar can offset the effect of high-glycemic foods (high glycemic foods are those primarily considered a simple carbohydrate) and reduce the spike in blood sugar after a meal. Vinegar has also been shown to help create a sense of satiety, thus reducing hunger—which can potentially contribute to weight loss.

Express yourself Boomer!

Appendix C

Resources and Support

Allergy and Asthma

National Institute of Allergy and Infectious Diseases (NIAID)
www.niaid.nih.org
NIAID Office of Communications and Government Relations
6610 Rockledge Drive, MSC 6612
Bethesda, MD 20892-6612
Toll-free: 866-284-4107
Phone: 301-496-5717
TDD: 800-877-8339
Fax: 301-402-3573

Asthma and Allergy Foundation (AAFA)
www.aafa.org
Asthma and Allergy Foundation of America
8201 Corporate Drive, Ste. 1000
Landover, MD 20785
Phone: 800-727-8462

Food Allergy and Anaphylaxis Network (FAAN)
www.foodallergy.org
11781 Lee Jackson Hwy., Ste. 160
Fairfax, VA 22033-3309
Phone: 800-929-4040
Fax: 703-691-2713

Arthritis

Arthritis Foundation
www.arthritis.org
P.O. Box 7669
Atlanta, GA 30357-0669
Toll-free: 800-283-7800

National Institute of Arthritis and Musculoskeletal and Skin Diseases (NIAMS)
Information Clearinghouse
National Institutes of Health
www.niams.nih.gov
AMS Circle
Bethesda, MD 20892-3675
Phone: 301-495-4484
Toll-free: 877-226-4267
TTY: 301–565–2966
Fax: 301-718-6366
Email: *NIAMSinfo@mail.nih.gov*

Bone Health

National Institutes of Health Osteoporosis and Related Bone Diseases
www.niams.nih.gov
AMS Circle
Bethesda, MD 20892-3676
Phone: 202-223-0344
Toll-free: 800-624-BONE
TTY: 202-466-4315
Fax: 202-293-2356
Email: *NIAMSBoneInfo@mail.nih.gov*

National Osteoporosis Foundation
www.nof.org
1150 17th Street NW, Ste. 850
Washington, DC 20036
Phone: 202-223.2226
Toll-free: 800-231-4222

Cancer

American Cancer Society
www.cancer.org
Phone: 800-227-2345

American Institute for Cancer Research (AICR)
www.aicr.org
1759 R Street, NW
Washington, DC 20009
Toll-free: 800-843-8114
Local: 202-328-7744 in D.C.
Fax: 202-328-7226
Email: *aicrweb@aicr.org*

National Cancer Institute (NCI)
www.cancer.gov
U.S. National Institutes of Health
6116 Executive Boulevard, Ste. 300
Bethesda, MD 20892-8322
Toll-free: 800-422-6237

Cardiovascular

American Heart Association
www.americanheart.org
7272 Greenville Ave.
Dallas, TX 75231
Toll-free: 800-242-8721
Spanish: 800-474-8483

National Heart Lung and Blood Institute (NHLBI) National Institutes of Health
www.nhlbi.nih.gov
NHLBI Health Information Center
P.O. Box 30105
Bethesda, MD 20824-0105
Phone: 301-592-8573
TTY: 240-629-3255
Fax: 240-629-3246

Celiac Disease and Digestive Health

American Gastroenterological Association
www.gastro.org
4930 Del Ray Avenue
Bethesda, MD 20814
Phone: (301) 654-2055
Fax: (301) 654-5920
Email: *member@gastro.org*

Canadian Celiac Association
www.celiac.ca
5170 Dixie Road, Suite 204
Mississauga ON L4W 1E3 Canada
Phone: 905-507-6208
Toll-free: 1-800-363-7296
Email: *info@celiac.ca*

Celiac Disease Foundation
www.celiac.org
13251 Ventura Blvd., Ste. 1
Studio City, CA 91604
Phone: 818-990-2354
Fax: 818-990-2379
Email: *cdf@celiac.org*

Gluten Intolerance Group of North America (GIG)
www.gluten.net
31214 124th Ave SE
Auburn, WA 98092-3667
Phone: 253-833-6655
Fax: 253-833-6675

National Digestive Diseases Information Clearinghouse (NIDDK)
www.digestive.niddk.nih.gov
2 Information Way
Bethesda, MD 20892–3570
Toll-free: 1–800–891–5389
TTY: 1–866–569–1162
Fax: 703–738–4929
Email: *nddic@info.niddk.nih.gov*

Consumer Health, Information, and Safety

American National Standards Institute (ANSI)
www.ansi.org
Washington, DC Headquarters
1819 L Street, NW, 6th Floor
Washington, DC 20036
Phone: 202-293-8020
Fax: 202-293-9287

Center for Disease Control and Prevention
www.cdc.gov
Division of Nutrition, Physical Activity and Obesity
4770 Buford Highway, NE, MS/K-24
Atlanta, GA 30341-3717
Toll-free: 800-232-4636
TTY: 888-232-6348
Email: *cdcinfo@cdc.gov*

Center for Science in the Public Interest
www.cspinet.org
1875 Connecticut Ave. NW, Ste. 300
Washington, DC 20009
Phone: 202-332-9110
Fax: 202-265-4954

FDA Medwatch
www.fda.gov/safety/medwatch/howtoreport/default.htm
MedWatch 5600 Fishers Lane
Rockville, MD 20852-9787
Phone: 888-332-1088
Fax: 800-332-0178

Federal Trade Commission (FTC)
ftc.gov/health
600 Pennsylvania Ave, NW
Washington, DC 20580
Phone: 202-326-2222
Toll-free: 877-382-4357
TTY: 1-866-653-4261

Food and Drug Administration (FDA)
www.fda.gov, www.cfsan.fda.gov
Center for Food Safety and Applied Nutrition
Food and Drug Administration
5100 Paint Branch Parkway
College Park, MD 20740
Toll-free: 888-723-3366

International Food Information Council Foundation
www.foodinsight.org
1100 Connecticut Avenue NW, Ste. 430
Washington, DC 20036
Phone: 202-296-6540
Email: *info@foodinsight.org*

National Center for Complementary and Alternative Medicine
www.nccam.nih.gov
National Institutes of Health
9000 Rockville Pike
Bethesda, Maryland 20892
Phone: 888-644-6226
TTY: 1-866-464-3615
Email: *info@nccam.nih.gov*

National Institute on Aging
www.nia.nih.gov
Building 31, Room 5C27
31 Center Drive, MSC 2292
Bethesda, MD 20892
Toll-free: 800-222-2225
Phone: 301-496-1752
TTY: 1-800-222-4225
Fax: 301-496-1072

National Sanitation Foundation International (NSF)
www.nsf.org
P.O. Box 130140
789 N. Dixboro Road
Ann Arbor, MI 48113-0140
Toll-free: 800-673-6275
Phone: 734-769-8010
Fax: 734-769-0109
Email: *info@nsf.org*

Office of Dietary Supplements
www.ods.od.nih.gov
National Institutes of Health
6100 Executive Blvd., Room 3B01, MSC 7517
Bethesda, MD 20892-7517
Phone: 301-435-2920
Fax: 301-480-1845
Email: *ods@nih.gov*

United States Department of Agriculture (USDA)
www.usda.gov
U.S. Department of Agriculture
1400 Independence Ave., S.W.
Washington, DC 20250
Phone: 202-720-2791

United States Department of Health and Human Services
www.healthfinder.gov
P.O. Box 1133
Washington, DC 20013-1133
Email: *healthfinder@nhic.org*

U.S. Pharmacopeia
www.usp.org
12601 Twinbrook Parkway
Rockville, Maryland 20852–1790
Toll-free: 800-227-8772
Phone: 301-881-0666

Dental

American Dental Association
www.ada.org
211 East Chicago Ave.
Chicago, IL 60611-2678
Phone: 312-440-2500

Diabetes

American Diabetes Association
www.diabetes.org
1701 North Beauregard Street
Alexandria, VA 22311
Toll-free: 800-342-2383

Eye Health

American Academy of Opthalmology
www.aao.org
P.O. Box 7424
San Francisco, CA 94120-7424
Phone: 415-561-8500
Fax: 415-561-8533

National Eye Institute
www.nei.nih.gov
National Eye Institute Information Office
31 Center Drive MSC 2510
Bethesda, MD 20892-2510
Phone: 301-496-5248
E-mail: *2020@nei.nih.gov*

Food and Nutrition Information

American Dietetic Association
www.eatright.org
120 S. Riverside Plaza, Ste. 2000
Chicago, IL 60606
Phone: 800-877-1600

Healthy Eating
www.mypyramid.gov
USDA Center for Nutrition Policy and Promotion
3101 Park Center Drive, Room 1034
Alexandria, VA 22302-1594
Phone: 1-888-779-7264
Email: *support@cnpp.usda.gov*

Genetic Testing and Research

Genova Diagnostics
www.gdx.net
63 Zillicoa Street
Asheville, NC 28801
Toll-free: 800-522-4762
Local: 828-253-0621

Interleukin Genetics Incorporated
www.ilgenetics.com
135 Beaver Street
Waltham, MA 02452
Phone: 781-398-0700
Fax: 781-398-0720

National Genome Research Institute
www.genome.gov
National Human Genome Research Institute
National Institutes of Health
Building 31, Room 4B09
31 Center Drive, MSC 2152
9000 Rockville Pike
Bethesda, MD 20892-2152
Phone: 301-402-0911
Fax: 301-402-2218

Lung Health

American Lung Association

www.lungusa.org
1301 Pennsylvania Ave., NW, Ste. 800
Washington, DC 20004
Phone: 212-315-8700
Helpline: 800-548-8252

Nanotechnology

National Nanotechnology Initiative

www.nano.gov
National Nanotechnology Coordination Office
4201 Wilson Blvd., Stafford II, Rm. 405
Arlington, VA 22230
Phone: 703-292-8626
Fax: 703-292-9312

Professional Associations

American Board of Physician Nutrition Specialists (ABPNS)

www.main.uab.edu/Sites/abpns/
American Board of Physician Nutrition Specialists
The University of Alabama at Birmingham
Community Health Services Building-19, Room 302
933 19th Street South
Birmingham, AL 35294-2041
Phone: 205-996-2513
Fax: 205-934-7438

American Chiropractic Organization

www.acatoday.org
1701 Clarendon Boulevard
Arlington, VA 22209
Phone: 703-276-8800
Fax: 703-243-2593
Email: *memberinfo@acatoday.org*

American Medical Association

www.ama.org
515 N. State Street
Chicago, IL 60654
Toll-free: 800-621-8335

American Osteopathic Association

www.osteopathic.org
142 East Ontario Street
Chicago, IL 60611
Toll-free: (800) 621-1773
Phone: 312-202-8000
Fax 312-202-8200

American Society of Exercise Physiologists (ASEP)

www.asep.org
c/o The College of St. Scholastica
1200 Kenwood Avenue
Duluth, MN 55811
Phone: 218 723 6297
Fax: 218 723 6472

American Society of Physical Therapists (APTA)

www.apta.org
American Physical Therapy Association
1111 North Fairfax Street
Alexandria, VA 22314-1488
Toll-free: 800-999-2782
Phone: 703-684-2782
TDD: 703-683-6748
Fax: 703-684-7343

Certification Board for Nutrition Specialists (CBNS)
www.cbns.org
300 S. Duncan Ave. Suite 225
Clearwater, FL 33755
Phone: 727- 446-6086
Fax: 727-446-6202

Clinical Nutrition Certification Board (CNCB)
www.cncb.org
Clinical Nutrition Certification Board
15280 Addison Road, Ste. 130
Addison, TX 75001
Phone: 972-250-2829
Fax: 972-250-0233

Council on Naturopathic Medical Education (CNME)
www.cnme.org
P. O. Box 178
Great Barrington, MA 01230
Phone: 413-528-8877

Skin Care

American Academy of Dermatology
www.aad.org

Sleep

American Sleep Association
www.americansleepassociation.org

National Heart, Lung, and Blood Institute (NHLBI)
www.nhlbi.nih.gov/sleep
National Center on Sleep Disorders Research
National Heart, Lung, and Blood Institute
National Institutes of Health
6705 Rockledge Drive, Ste. 6022
Bethesda, MD 20892–7993
Phone: 301–435–0199
Fax: 301–480–3451
Email: *ncsdr@nih.gov*

Notes

Chapter 1. Our Generation

A Global Effect

1. Heller, L., "Global strategy called in for obesity battle," *http://www.foodnavigator-usa.com/news/ng.asp?n=67771&m=1FNU517&c=eyenaejorjrly* ... Accessed May 17, 2006.

2. *Rocky Mountain News*, August 19, 2006: 26A

3. Rundle, R. L., "Health-care costs for obesity top those related to smoking," *http://www.karlloren.com/diet/p69.htm* ... Accessed March 12, 2002.

4. Fletcher, A., "Commissioner warns of obesity related economic meltdown," *http://www.nutraingredients.com/news/printNewsBis.asp?id=67691* ... Accessed May 15, 2006.

An Era in Eating

5. "Beverage intake in the United States. Why a beverage panel? You are what you drink and we are drinking far too many calories from beverages," *http://www.cpc.unc.edu/projects/beverage?makePrintable=1&style=1119* ... Accessed February 21, 2008.

6. Murray, M., Pizzorno, J., Pizzorno, L., *The Encyclopedia of Healing Foods* (New York: Atria Books, 2005), 784-5.

New Science

Nutritional Genomics

7. DeBusk, R., Joffe, Y., Fogarty, C., Bischoff, B., "Understanding nutrigenomics and its practical applications," *Nutrition in Complementary Care*, Spring (2006);8 (4): 61.

8. See note 7 above.

9. "President Bush signs the genetic information nondiscrimination act of 2008," National Human Genome Research Institute, *http://www.genome.gov/27026050* ... Accessed June 15, 2008.

Nanotechnology

10. "What is nanotechnology?" *http://www.nano.gov/html/facts/whatIsNano.html* ... Accessed January 18, 2010.

11. See note 10 above.

12. Schmipf, S., "The Future of Medicine: Megatrends in Healthcare that will improve the quality of your life," (Nashville: Thomas Nelson, 2007), 112.

13. Nickols-Richardson, S. M., "Nanotechnology: Implications for food and nutrition professionals," *J Am Diet Assoc* (2007);107(9):1494-1497.

14. Powell, M. C., Kanarek, M. S., "Nanomaterial health effects—Part 2: Uncertainties and recommendations for the future," *WMJ* (2006); 105:18-23.

15. See note 10 above.

16. See note 13 above.

17. See note 12 above.

18. See note 13 above.

19. See note 14 above.

20. Boyce, B., "Knowing nanotech is knowing the future of food and nutrition," *J Am Diet Assoc* (2009);109(8):1332-1335.

21. See note 12 above.

22. See note 13 above.

23. See note 20 above.

24. Nanotechnology fact sheet, *http://www.nsf.gov/news/news_summ.jsp?cntn_id=100602* ... Accessed January 24, 2010.

25. See note 10 above.
26. See note 21 above.

Chapter 2. Buyer Be Aware

Never Underestimate the Power of Advertising

1. Austin, S., "Temptation television," *Self*, November, 2006:157.

The Promise of Eternal Youth

2. Boyles, S., "New warnings for women taking HRT estrogen-only therapy linked to ovarian cancer," *http://www.webmd.com/menopause/news/20020716/new-warnings-for-women-taking-hrt-news* ... Accessed July 16, 2002.

Types of Medicine and Those Who Practice It

3. "Qualifications of a registered dietitian," *http://www.eatright.org/HealthProfessionals/content.aspx?id=6857* ... Accessed April 4, 2010.
4. "What is a dietetic technician, registered?" *http://www.eatright.org/HealthProfessionals/content.aspx?id=6861* ... Accessed April 4, 2010.
5. "Certified nutritionist," *http://www.ahsu.edu/cn.html* ... Accessed January 12, 2010.
6. "What is a nutritionist?" *http://www.cbns.org/* ... Accessed December 3, 2009.
7. "Clinical nutrition certification board," *http://www.cncb.org/* ... Accessed December 3, 2009.
8. "Credentialing for physician nutrition specialist," *http://main.uab.edu/Sites/abpns/pns/46530/* ... Accessed December 3, 2009.
9. "Chiropractors," United States Department of Labor, *http://www.bls.gov/oco/ocos071.htm* ... Accessed January 1, 2010.
10. "What is CAM?" *http://nccam.nih.gov/health/whatiscam/* ... Accessed January 2007.
11. See note 10 above.
12. "An introduction to naturopathy," *http://nccam.nih.gov/health/naturopathy/* ... Accessed January 15, 2007.
13. See note 12 above.
14. See note 12 above.

Chapter 3. Supplements, Antioxidants and Food Allergies

The Case for Supplements

1. "What is creatine?" *http://men.webmd.com/creatine* ... Accessed February 13, 2010.

2. Buch, L. J., "Fueling the older athlete for triumph," *http://www.denverpost.com/headlines/ci_10517198* ... Accessed September 22, 2008.

3. Volek, J. S., "Creatine: The next anti-aging supplement?" *http://www.nutritionexpress.com/article+index/authors/jeff+s+volek+phd+rd+facn/showarticle.aspx?articleid=907* ... Accessed February 13, 2010.

4. "Fish and omega-3 fatty acids," *http://www.americanheart.org/presenter.jhtml?identifier=4632* ... Accessed January 1, 2009.

5. Peckenpaugh, N., *Nutrition Essentials and Diet Therapy, 10th Ed.,* (Amsterdam: Elsevier, 2007), 56.

6. Ranjekar, P. K., Hinge, A., Hedge, M. V., Ghate, M., Kale, A., Sitasawad, S., Wagh, U. V., "Decreased antioxidant enzymes and membrane essential polyunsaturated fatty acids in schizophrenia and bipolar mood disorder patients," *Psychiatry Res* (2003);121(2):109-122.

7. Skarnulis, L., "Arthritis diets & supplements: Do they work?" *http://www.webmd.com/osteoarthritis/guide/arthritis-diets-supplements?page=2* ... Accessed September 23, 2005.

8. *Nutrition Business Journal*, San Diego, 1998.

9. "FDA's progress with dietary supplements," *http://www.fda.gov/NewsEvents/Testimony/ucm115229.htm* ... Accessed July 25, 2009.

10. "Regulatory framework of DSHEA of 1994," *http://www.fda.gov/NewsEvents/Testimony/ucm115163.htm* ... Accessed June 25, 2009.

11. "Overview of dietary supplements: What is a dietary supplement?" *http://www.fda.gov/Food/DietarySupplements/ConsumerInformation/ucm110417.htm* ... Accessed April 4, 2010.

12. See note 11 above.

13. See note 11 above.

14. "Nutrition education and labeling act (NLEA) requirements (8/94-2/95)," *http://www.fda.gov/ICECI/Inspections/InspectionGuides/ucm074948.htm#LABEL REVIEW* ... Accessed February 6, 2010.

15. See note 14 above.

16. "Guidance for industry: Food labeling; nutrient content claims; definition for 'high potency' and definition for 'antioxidant' for use in nutrient content claims for dietary supplements and conventional foods; small entity compliance guide," *http://www.fda.gov/Food/GuidanceCompliance RegulatoryInformation/GuidanceDocuments/FoodLabelingNutrition/ucm06 3064.htm* ... Accessed April 4, 2010.

17. See note 11 above.

18. "US dietary supplements often contaminated: Report," *http:// www.lifescript.com/Health/News/Reuters/2010/08/03/US_dietary_ supplements_often contaminated_report.aspx?utm_campaign=2010-08- 05-57074&utm_source=healthy-advantage&utm_medium=email& utm_content=healthy-news-bites_US%20dietary%20supplement&From NL=1&sc_date=20100805T000000* ... Accessed August 22, 2010.

19. "A dirty dozen list of supplements consumers should avoid," *http://pressroom.consumerreports.org/pressroom/2010/08/yonkers-ny-a-new- investigation-in-the-september-issue-of-consumer-reports-and-available- online-at-wwwconsumerreportshea.html* ... Accessed August 22, 2010.

Can Supplements Help Extend Life?

20. Stibich, M., "Telomeres and aging-understanding cellular aging," <a href="http://longevity.about.com/od/researchandmedicine/p/telomeres. htm">http://longevity.about.com/od/researchandmedicine/p/telomeres.htm </a> ... Accessed September 5, 2009.

21. Daniells, S., "Tea consumers may have younger biological age," *http://www.nutraingredients.com/content/view/print/257355* ... Accessed August 30, 2009.

22. Chan, R., Woo, J., Suen, E., Leung, J., Tang, N., "Chinese tea consumption is associated with longer telomere length in elderly Chinese men," *Brit J Nutr* doi:10.1017/S0007114509991383.

23. Farzaneh-Far, R., Lin, J., Epel, E. S., Harris, W. S., Blackburn, E. H., Whooley, M. A., "Association of marine omega-3 fatty acid levels with telomeric aging in patients with coronary heart disease," *JAMA* (2010) 303; (3): 250-257.

24. "Introduction to omega-3," *http://www.dhaomega3.org/Overview/ Introduction-to-Omega-3* ... Accessed October 6, 2010.

The Importance of Vitamin D

25. Holick, M. F., "Sunlight and vitamin D for bone health and prevention of autoimmune diseases, cancers, and cardiovascular disease," *Am J Clin Nutr* (2004); 80(suppl):1678S-88S.

26. "Vitamin D deficiency common in patients with IBD, chronic liver disease: Vitamin D replacement may be necessary to reverse deficiency-related bone loss," *American College of Gastroenterology*, October 6, 2008. *http://www.acg.gi.org/media/releases/2008am/ACG08VitaminDDefi ciency.pdf*

27. Plotnikoff, G. A., Quigley, J. M., "Prevalence of severe hypovitaminosis D in patients with persistent, nonspecific musculoskeletal pain," *Mayo Clinic Proc* (2003); 78:1463-70.

28. Holick, M. F., "Vitamin D deficiency: What a pain it is," *Mayo Clin Proc* (2003); 78:1457-9.

29. Glerup, H., Middelsen, K., Poulsen, L., et al., "Hypovitaminosis D myopathy without biochemical signs of osteolmalacia bone involvement," *Calcif Tissue Int* (2000); 66:419-24.

30. Munger, K. L., Zhang, S. M., O'Reilly, E., Herman, M. A., Olek, M. J., Willet, W. C., Ascherio, A., "Vitamin D intake and incidence of multiple sclerosis," *Neurology* (2004); 62:60-65.

31. Cruz, J., Cosman, F., Cantorna, M. T., "Cytokine profile in patients with multiple sclerosis following vitamin D supplementation," *J Neuroimmunol.*(2003); 134:128-132.

32. Lu, L., Pan, A., Hu, F. B., Franco, O. H., Li, H., Li, X., Yang, X., Chen, Y., Yu, Z., Lin, X., "Plasma 25-hydroxyvitamin D concentration and metabolic syndrome among middle-aged and elderly Chinese," *Diabetes Care* doi 10.2337/dc09-0209.

33. Hoogendijk, W. J. G., Lips, P., Dik, M. G., Deeg, D. J. H., Beekman, A. T. F., Penninx, B. W. J. H., "Depression is associated with decreased 25-Hydroxyvitamin D and increased parathyroid hormone levels in older adults," *Archives of General Psychiatry* (2008);65(5):508-512.

34. Dietary supplement fact sheet: Vitamin D, *http://ods.od.nih.gov/ factsheets/vitamind.asp* ... Accessed September 1, 2010.

35. Brannon, P. M., Yetley, E. A., Bailey, R. L., Picciano, M. F., Overview of the conference "Vitamin D and Health in the 21st century: An update," *Am J Clin Nutr* (2008); 88(suppl):483S-90S.

36. Shelke, K., "Vitamins take the lead with consumers," Food Processing.com *http://www.foodprocessing.com/articles/2009/wellnessfebruaryvitamins.html?page=print* ... Accessed April 13, 2009.

37. Institute of Medicine, Food and Nutrition Board, "Dietary Reference Intakes: Calcium, Phosphorus, Magnesium, Vitamin D, and Fluoride," (Washington, DC: National Academy Press, 1997).

38. Cranney, C., Horsely, T., O' Donnell, S., Weiler, H., Ooi, D., Atkinson, S., et al., "Effectiveness and safety of vitamin D. Evidence Report/ Technology Assessment No. 158 prepared by the University of Ottawa Evidence-based Practice Center under Contract No. 290-02.0021," AHRQ Publication No. 07-E013. Rockville, MD: Agency for Healthcare Research and Quality, 2007. [*PubMed abstract*]

39. Goldring, S. R., Krane, S., Avioli, L. V., "Disorders of calcification: Osteomalacia and rickets," In: DeGroot, L. J., Besser, M., Burger, H. G., Jameson, J. L., Loriaux, D.L., Marshall, J.C., et al., eds. *Endocrinology*, 3rd ed. (Philadelphia: WB Saunders, 1995):1204-27.

40. Holick, M. F., "Resurrection of vitamin D deficiency and rickets," *J Clin Investigation* (2006);116(8):2062-2072.

41. Malone, R. W., Kessenich, C., "Vitamin D deficiency: Implications across the lifespan," *J Nurse Pract* (2008); 4(6):448-456.

42. Hayes, C. E., Hashold, F. E., Spach, K. M., Pederson, L. B., "The immunological functions of the vitamin D endocrine system," *Cell Mol Biol* (2003); 49:277-300. [*PubMed abstract*]

43. See note 36 above.

44. See note 34 above.

45. See note 25 above.

46. See note 41 above.

47. Holick, M. F., "Vitamin D deficiency," *N Engl J Med* (2007);357: 266-281.

48. See note 34 above.

49. See note 35 above.

50. DeLuca, H. F., "Overview of general physiologic features and functions of vitamin D," *Am J Clin Nutr* (2004);80:1689S-96S. [*PubMed abstract*]

51. See note 34 above.

52. See note 35 above.

53. Holick, M. F., "Vitamin D benefits for bone health and beyond," *www.beveraginstitute.org* ... Accessed April 14, 2009.

54. See note 36 above.

55. See note 38 above.

56. See note 34 above.

57. *http://www.nof.org/aboutosteoporosis/prevention/vitamind.*

58. See note 34 above.

59. See note 37 above.

60. See note 53 above.

61. Oveson, L., Brot, C., Jakobsen, J., "Food contents and biological activity of 25-hydroxyvitamin D: A vitamin D metabolite to be reckoned with?" *Ann Nutr Metab* (2003);47:107-13.

62. See note 34 above.

63. Beelman, R., Kalaras, M., "Post-harvest vitamin D enrichment of fresh mushroom," (2009) http://mushroominfo.com/wp-content/uploads/PSU_Vit_D_Mushroom_Study.pdf ... Accessed April 3, 2011.

64. Outila, T. A., Mattila, P. H., Piironen, V. I., Lamberg-Allardt, C. J. E., "Bioavailability of vitamin D from wild edible mushrooms (Cantharellus tubaeformis) as measured with a human bioassay," *Am J Clin Nutr* (1999);69:95-8. [*PubMed abstract*]

65. See note 34 above.

66. See note 37 above.

67. See note 63 above.

68. Calvo, M. S., Whiting, S. J., Barton, C. N., "Vitamin D fortification in the United States and Canada: Current status and data needs," *Am J Clin Nutr* (2004);80:1710S-6S. [*PubMed abstract*]

69. See note 25 above.

70. See note 34 above.

71. Vitamin D Council, "Sunshine and your health," *http://www.vitamindcouncil.org/* ... Accessed April 28, 2009.

72. See note 34 above.

73. See note 47 above.

74. Holick, M. F., "Vitamin D: The underappreciated D-lightful hormone that is important for skeletal and cellular health," *Curr Opin Endocrinol Diabetes* (2002);9:87-98.

75. See note 25 above.

76. See note 25 above.

77. See note 34 above.

78. See note 38 above.

79. See note 53 above.

80. See note 34 above.

81. Wharton, B., Bishop, N., "Rickets," *Lancet* (2003);362:1389-400. [*PubMed abstract*]

82. See note 47 above.

83. See note 79 above.

84. See note 25 above.

85. See note 34 above.

86. See note 53 above.

87. Clemens, T. L., Henderson, S. L., Adams, J. S., Holick, M. F., "Increased skin pigment reduces the capacity of skin to synthesize vitamin D_3," *Lancet* (1982);1:74-6.

88. See note 34 above.

89. Wolpowitz, D., Gilchrest, B. A., "The vitamin D questions: How much do you need and how should you get it?" *J Am Acad Dermatol* (2006);54:301-17. [*PubMed abstract*]

90. International Agency for Research on Cancer Working Group on ultraviolet (UV) light and skin cancer, "The association of use of sunbeds with cutaneous malignant melanoma and other skin cancers: A systematic revue," *Int J Cancer* (2006);120:1116-22. [*PubMed abstract*]

91. See note 34 above.

92. Lo, C. W., Paris, P. W., Clemens, T. L., Nolan, J., Holick, M. F., "Vitamin D absorption in healthy subjects and in patients with intestinal malabsorption syndromes," *Am J Clin Nutr* (1985);42:644-49. [*PubMed abstract*]

93. Holick, M. F., "Vitamin D," In: Shils, M. E., Shike, M., Ross, A. C., Caballero, B., Cousins, R. J., eds., *Modern Nutrition in Health and Disease, 10th ed.* (Philadelphia: Lippincott, Williams & Wilkins, 2006).

94. Wortsman, J., Matsuoka, L. Y., Chen, T. C., Lu, Z., Holick, M. F., "Decreased bioavailability of vitamin D in obesity," *Am J Clin Nutr* (2000);72:690-3. [*PubMed abstract*]

95. Vilarrasa, N., Maravall, J., Estepa, A., Sanchez, R., Masdevall, C., Navarro, M.A., et al., "Low 25-hydroxyvitamin D concentrations in obese

women: Their clinical significance and relationship with anthropometric and body composition variables," *J Endocrinol Invest* (2007);30:653-8. [*PubMed abstract*]

96. Malone, M., "Recommended nutritional supplements for bariatric surgery patients," *Ann Pharmacother* (2008);42:1851-8. [*PubMed abstract*]

97. See note 37 above.

98. See note 34 above.

99. Jones, G., "Pharmacokinetics of vitamin D toxicity," *Am J Clin Nutr* (2008);88:582S-6S. [*PubMed abstract*]

100. See note 34 above.

101. See note 99 above.

102. Chung, M., Balk, E. M., Brendel, M., Ip, S., Lau, J., Lee, J., et al.," Vitamin D and calcium: A systematic review of health outcomes," Evidence Report/Technology Assessment No. 183, prepared by the Tufts Evidence-based Practice Center under Contract No. 290-2007-10055-I. AHRQ Publication No. 09-E015. (Rockville, MD: Agency for Healthcare Research and Quality, 2009).

103. Favus, M. J., Christakos, S., *Primer on the Metabolic Bone Diseases and Disorders of Mineral Metabolism. 3rd ed.* (Philadelphia: Lippincott-Raven, 1996).

104. Jackson, R. D., LaCroix, A. Z., Gass, M., Wallace, R. B., Robbins, J., Lewis, C.E., et al., "Calcium plus vitamin D supplementation and the risk of fractures," *N Engl J Med* (2006);354:669-83. [*PubMed abstract*]

105. "NOF recommendations for vitamin D," http://www.nof.org/aboutosteoporosis/prevention/vitamind ... Accessed April 13, 2011.

106. Hathcock, J. N., Shao, A., Vieth, R., Heaney, R., "Risk assessment for vitamin D," *Am J Clin Nutr* (2007);85:6-18. [*PubMed abstract*]

107. Buckley, L. M., Leib, E. S., Cartularo, K. S., Vacek, P. M., Cooper, S. M., "Calcium and vitamin D_3 supplementation prevents bone loss in the spine secondary to low-dose corticosteroids in patients with rheumatoid arthritis. A randomized, double-blind, placebo-controlled trial," *Ann Intern Med* (1996);125:961-8. [*PubMed abstract*]

108. Lukert, B. P., Raisz, L.G., "Glucocorticoid-induced osteoporosis: Pathogenesis and management," *Ann Intern Med* (1990);112:352-64. [*PubMed abstract*]

Prebiotics, Probiotics and Immunity

109. International Food Information Council Foundation, "Functional foods fact sheet: Probiotics and prebiotics." "Probiotics - Topic overview," *http://www.foodinsight.org/Resources/Detail.aspx?topic=Functional_Foods_ Fact_Sheet_Probiotics_and_Prebiotics* … Accessed April 12, 2010.

110. Gibson, G. R., "Dietary modulation of the human gut microflora using the prebiotics oligofructose and inulin," *Am Society Nutr Sci* (1999);129:1438S-1441S.

111. Duyff, R. L., *American Dietetic Association Complete Food and Nutrition Guide, 2nd Ed.* (Hoboken: John Wiley & Sons, Inc., 2002), 111.

112. See note 109 above.

113. See note 111 above.

114. "Probiotics-Topic interview," *http://www.webmd.com/diet/tc/ probiotics-topic-overview* … Accessed April 12, 2010.

115. See note 109 above.

116. See note 111 above.

117. See note 114 above.

118. Saavendra, J. M., Tschemia, A., "Human studies with probiotics and prebiotics: Clinical implications," *British J Nutr* 2002;87:S241-S246.

119. Cummings, J. H., Macfarlane, G. T., "A study of fructo oligosac-charides in the prevention of travelers' diarrhea," *Aliment Pharmacol Ther* (2001);15(8):1139-1145.

Antioxidants

120. Weil, A., "The healthiest way to eat," *Self,* November, 2005: 98.

121. "Antioxidants," *http://www.nlm.nih.gov/medlineplus/antioxi-dants.html* … Accessed January 15, 2008.

122. "Antioxidants-Topic Overview," *http://www.webmd.com/diet/tc/ Antioxidants-Topic-Overview* … Accessed January 15, 2008.

123. See note 122 above.

124. "Antioxidants and cancer prevention: Fact sheet," *http://www. cancer.gov/cancertopics/factsheet/prevention/antioxidants* … Accessed January 16, 2008.

125. "Institute of medicine releases DRI's for antioxidants and related compounds," *J Am Diet Assoc* Vol. 98(12):1411.

126. See note 111 above, p. 89.

127. See note 122 above.

Don't Forget the Herbs and Spices

128. "Food Facts," Dole Nutrition Institute, *http://www.dole.com/L%20-%20R/tabid/1000/Default.aspx* ... Accessed August 10, 2010.

129. Grotto, D., *101 Foods That Could Save Your Life* (New York: Bantam Dell, 2007), 225-228.

130. Aydin, S., Basaran, A. A., Basaran, N., "Modulating effects of thyme and its major ingredients on oxidative DNA damage in human lymphocytes," *J Agriculture and Food Chemistry* (2005); 53:1299-1305.

131. Hotta, M., Nakata, R., Katsukawa, M., Hori, K., Takahashi, S., Inoue, H. "Carvacrol, a component of thyme oil, activates PPARalpha and gamma and suppresses COX-2 expression," *J Lipid Research* (2009); 51:132-139.

132. Moss, M., Cook, J., Wasnes, K., Duckett, P., "Aromas of rosemary and lavender essential oils on test-taking anxiety among graduate nursing students," *Holistic Nursing Practice* (2009);23:88-93.

133. Takaki, I., Bersani-Amado, L. E., Vendruscolo, A., Sartpretto, S. M., Diniz, S. P., Bersani-Amado, C. A., Cuman, R. K., "Anti-inflammatory and antinociceptive effects of rosmarinus officinalis L. essential oil in experimental animal models," *J of Medicinal Food* (2008); 11:741-746.

134. See note 128 above.

135. See note 128 above.

136. See note 129 above.

137. See note 129 above, pp. 334-338.

138. Neville, K., "Spice up your health: Some seasonings carry anti-oxidant benefits as well as wonderful flavor," *http://www.chicagotribune.com/features/food/chi-0609130054sep13,1,179195.story?coll* ... Accessed September 14, 2006.

139. See note 138 above.

140. Khan, A., Safdar, M., Khan, M., Khattak, K., Anderson, R., "Cinnamon improves glucose and lipids of people with type 2 diabetes," *Diabetes Care* (2003); 26 (12):3215-3218.

141. Khan, A., Safdar, M., Khan, M., "Effect of various doses of

cinnamon on lipid profile in diabetic individuals," *Pakistan Journal of Nutrition* (2003); 2(5):312-319.

142. See note 129 above, pp. 147-149.

143. Grzanna, R., Phan, P., Polotsky, A., Lindmark, L., Frondoza, C. G., "Ginger extract inhibits beta-amyloid peptide-induced cytokine and chemokine expression in cultured THP-1 monocytes," *J Altern Complement Med* (2004) 10(6):1009-13.

Changes That Occur When Cooking Food

144. *http://www.cancer.org/docroot/NWS/content/NWS_1_1x_Acry-lamide_Cancer_Risk_Not_Known_For_Humans_Experts_Say.asp* ... Accessed May 3, 2005.

145. "Plan to cut cancer risk in fried foods," *http://news.smh.com.au/national/plan-to-cut-cancer-risk-in-fried-foods-20070812-su9.html* ... Accessed August 13, 2007.

146. See note 145 above.

147. Daniells, S., "Hydrocolloids may inhibit acrylamide formation," *http://www.foodnavigator-usa.com/Science-Nutrition/Hydrocolloids-may-inhibit-acrylamide-formation* ... Accessed August 20, 2010.

148. "Barbecuing made healthy. A backyard chef's guide to healthy grilling," *http://www.cancer.org/docroot/NWS/content/NWS_1_1x_Barbecuing_Made_Healthy.asp* ... Accessed December 19, 2007.

149. "Give burgers a boost this summer. Veggies, fruits, add flavor, nutrients to cookouts," *http://www.cancer.org/docroot/NWS/content/NWS_2_1x_Give_Burgers_a_Boost_This_Summer.asp* ... Accessed December 19, 2007.

150. "Detailed guide: stomach cancer. What are the risk factors for stomach cancer?" *http://www.cancer.org/docroot/CRI/content/CRI_2_4_2X_What_are_the_risk_factors_for_stomach_cancer_40.asp* ... Accessed December 19, 2007.

151. Daniells, S., "Antioxidant-rich spice mix shows potential for heart health," *http://www.foodnavigator.com/Science-Nutrition/Antioxidant-rich-spice-mix-shows-potential-for-heart-health* ... Accessed April 18, 2010.

152. See note 151 above.

153. Lord, M., "Healthy grill skills," *Self,* August (2008):78.

154. "Spicing the meat also cuts the cancer risk, research suggests." *http://www.sciencedaily.com/releases/2010/05/100518105801.htm* … Accessed June 30, 2010.

Food Allergies, Sensitivities, and Intolerances

155. "Food allergies: What you need to know," *http://www.fda.gov/Food/ResourcesForYou/Consumers/ucm079311.htm* … Accessed March 27, 2010.

156. See note 155 above.

157. What is food allergy?" *http://www.niaid.nih.gov/topics/foodAllergy/understanding/Pages/whatIsIt.aspx*… Accessed November 19, 2010.

158. Arshad, S. H., Bahna, S. L., Beck, L. A., Byrd-Bredbenner, C., Camargo, C. A., Eichenfield, L., Furuta, G. T., Hanifin, J. M., Jones, C., Kraft, M., Levy, B. D., Lieberman, P., Luccioli, S., McCall, K. M., Schneider, L. C., Simon, R. A., Simons, F. E. R., Teach, S. J., Yawn, B. P. "Guidelines for the diagnosis and management of food allergy in the United States: Report of the NIAID-Sponsored expert panel," *J Allergy and Clinical Immunology,* (2010);126 (6):S1-S58.

159. See note 157 above.

160. Jyonouchi, H. "Non-IgE mediated food allergy," *Inflamm Allergy Drug Targets,* 2008;7(3):173-80.

161. Chehade, M. "IgE and non-IgE-mediated food allergy: Treatment in 2007," *Curr Opin Allergy Clin Immunol* 2007;7(3):264-268.

161. "Food allergy: Diagnosis." *http://www.niaid.nih.gov/topics/foodAllergy/understanding/Pages/diagnosis.aspx*... Accessed February 12, 2011.

162. See note 158 above.

163. See note 161 above.

164. See note 158 above.

165. "Preventing and treating a food allergy," *http://www.niaid.nih.gov/TOPICS/FOODALLERGY/UNDERSTANDING/Pages/treatment.aspx#Treat,* Accessed February 12, 2011.

166. See note 158 above.

167. "Food allergies: What you need to know," *http://www.fda.gov/Food/ResourcesForYou/Consumers/ucm079311.htm* … Accessed February 12, 2011.

168. See note 167 above.

169. See note 165 above.

170. See note 157 above.

171. Bareuther, C. M., "Exploring testing options for delayed hyper-sensitivities," *Today's Dietitian,* January, 2009:20-22.

172. Interview with Jan Patenaude, RD, April 9, 2010.

173. See note 171 above.

174. Bulhoes, A. C., Goldani, H. A. S., Oliveira, F. S., et al., "Correlation between lactose absorption and the C/T-13910 and G/A-22018 mutations of the lactase-phlorizin hydrolase [LCT] gene in adult-type hypollactasia," *Braz J Med Biol Res* (2007);40(11):1441-1446.

175. Patenaude, J., "Is your food making you sick?" Signet Diagnostic Corporation, 2005-2006.

176. See note 172 above.

177. See note 172 above.

178. See note 174 above.

179. Cell Systems, Ltd., ALCAT food and chemical sensitivity test. *www.alcat.com* ... Accessed March 28, 2010.

180. See note 175 above.

181. See note 172 above.

182. See note 171 above.

183. "Lifestyle eating and performance," *http://www.forresthealth.com/leap-mrt-food-allergy-test.html* ... Accessed March 27, 2010.

184. See note 174 above.

185. See note 179 above.

186. See note 174 above.

187. See note 179 above.

188. See note 175 above.

189. See note 172 above.

190. See note 171 above.

191. See note 183 above.

192. See note 172 above.

Chapter 4. Food

Label Reading

1. Duyff, R. L., *American Dietetic Association Complete Food and Nutrition Guide, 2nd Ed.* (Hoboken:John Wiley & Sons, Inc., 2002), 120-125.

2. "Dietary guidance for Americans 2010," *http://www.health.gov/dietary =guidelines/dga2010/DietaryGuidelines2010.pdf* … Accessed February 16, 2012.

3. See note 1 above, p.83.

Safe Food Handling

4. *http://www.cdc.gov/ncidod/dbmd/diseaseinfo/foodborneinfections_g.htm#howmanycases* … Accessed February 15, 2011.

5. Scharff, R. L.,"Health related costs from foodborne illness in the United States. Produce Safety Project," March 3, 2010, p. 1. *http://www.producesafetyproject.org/admin/assets/files/Health-Related-Foodborne-Illness-Costs-Report.pdf-1.pdf*

6. See note 4 above.

7. "Refrigerate promptly below 40°F," *http://www.homefoodsafety.org/pages/4tips/tip4.jsp* Accessed August 21, 2010.

8. See note 7 above.

9. "Cook to proper temperatures," *http://www.homefoodsafety.org/pages/4tips/tip3.jsp* … Accessed August 21, 2010.

Chapter 5. Making Changes

The Dilemma of Dieting

1. "Slim differences in weight-loss plans," Tufts University Health & Nutrition Letter, October (2007); 25(8):3.

Thoughts and Beliefs

2. Hales, D., "We're changing the way we eat," *Parade*, 11/12/2006:4.

Chapter 6. Back to the Basics

Body Weight

1. "According to waist circumference," *http://www.nhlbi.nih.gov/guidelines/obesity/e_txtbk/txgd/4142.htm* … Accessed August 10, 2010.

2. "What does the latest research mean to you?" *http://www.tuftshealthletter.com/ShowArticle.aspx?rowId=114* … Accessed August 22, 2010.

3. Zelman, K., "The truth about belly fat," *http://www.webmd.com/diet/features/the-truth-about-belly-fat* … Accessed August 10, 2010.

4. "Aim for a healthy weight," National Heart, Lung and Blood Institute, *http://www.nhlbi.nih.gov/health/public/heart/obesity/lose_wt/* … Accessed February 20, 2008.

5. "How to prevent and control risk disease factors," *http://www.nhlbi.nih.gov/health/dci/Diseases/hd/hd_prevention.html* … Accessed August 23, 2010.

Daily Caloric Requirements

6. Duyff, R. L., *American Dietetic Association Complete Food and Nutrition Guide, 2nd Ed.* (Hoboken: John Wiley & Sons, Inc., 2002), 26.

7. Peckenpaugh, N., *Nutrition Essentials and Diet Therapy, 10th Ed.* (Amsterdam: Elsevier, 2007), 52.

8. See note 6 above.

Protein

9. See note 6 above, pp. 500-501.

10. See note 6 above, pp. 14, 15, 25, 484.

11. See note 7 above, p. 48.

12. See note 7 above, p. 51.

13. "Protein," *http://www.cdc.gov/nutrition/everyone/basics/protein.html?debugMode=false* … Accessed September 5, 2010.

14. See note 13 above.

15. Conolly-Schoonen, J., "Dietary protein intake differences based on activity level," *http://www.medscape.com/viewarticle/414351* … Accessed April 7, 2010.

16. Chernoff, R., "Protein and older adults," *J Am Coll Nutr* (2004); 23(suppl):627S-630S.

17. See note 7 above.

18. See note 6 above pp. 14, 15, 25, 484.

19. Layman, D. K., Boileau, R. A., Erickson, D. J., Painter, J. E., Shiue, H., Sather, C., Christou, D. D., "A reduced ratio of dietary carbohydrate to protein improves body composition and blood lipid profiles during weight loss in adult women," *J Nutr* (2003);133:411-417.

20. Piatti, P. M., Monti, F., Fermo, I., Baruffaldi, L., Masser, R., Santambrogio, G., Librenti, M. C., Galli-Kienle, M., Pontiroli, A. E., Pozza, G., "Hypocaloric high-protein diet improves glucose oxidation and spares lean body mass: Comparison to hypocaloric high-carbohydrate diet," *Metabolism* (1994);43:1481-1487.

21. Layman, D. K., Evans, E., Baum, J. I., Seyler, J., Erickson, D. J., Boileau, R. A., "Dietary protein and exercise have additive effects on body composition during weight loss in adult women," *J Nutr* (2005);135:1903-1910.

22. See note 6 above, pp. 14, 15, 25, 484.

23. See note 7 above, p. 48.

24. See note 7 above, p. 51.

25. See note 13 above.

26. See note 16 above.

27. See note 19 above.

28. See note 20 above.

29. See note 21 above.

30. See note 6 above, pp. 500-501.

31. See note 12 above, p. 51.

32. See note 6 above, p. 501.

33. See note 13 above.

Carbohydrates

34. See note 6 above, pp. 481-483.

35. "Choose carbohydrates wisely," *http://www.csrees.usda.gov/nea/food/pdfs/hhs_facts_carbohydrates.pdf* ... Accessed April 7, 2010.

36. See note 6 above, pp. 481-483.

37. See note 6 above, pp. 481-483.

38. "Carbohydrates," *http://www.cdc.gov/nutrition/everyone/basics/carbs.html#Simple Carbohydrates* ... Accessed April 5, 2010.

39. See note 6 above, pp. 481-483

40. See note 6 above, pp. 481-483.

41. "Dietary guidelines for Americans," *http://www.health.gov/dietary guidelines/dga2005/document/pdf/DGA2005.pdf* p. 49 ... Accessed April 5, 2010.

42. See note 6 above, pp. 481-483.

43. See note 35 above.

44. See note 6 above, pp. 481-483.

45. Halliday, J., "Low-fat better for mood than low-carb: Study," http://www.nutraingredients.com/content/view/print/267303 ... Accessed November 15, 2009.

46. Brinkworth, G., Buckley, J., Noakes, M., Clifton, P., Wilson, C., "Mood improves on low-fat but not low-carb diet plan." *Archives of Internal Medicine* 2009; 169(20):1873-1880. *http://www.newswise.com/articles/mood-improves-on-low-fat-but-not-low-carb-diet-plan.*

47. Bouchez, C., "Recognizing the symptoms of depression serotonin: 9 questions and answers," *http://www.webmd.com/depression/recognizing-depression-symptoms/serotonin?page=2&print=true* ... Accessed November 15, 2009.

48. See note 45 above.

49. See note 46 above.

50. See note 47 above.

51. See note 6 above, pp. 481-483.

52. See note 38 above.

Fat

53. See note 6 above, pp. 51-54.

54. "Fats: how to enjoy your food and be healthy too!" *http://www.foodinsight.org/Content/6/fatstipsheet.pdf* ... Accessed April 6, 2010.

55. "Saturated fats," *http://www.americanheart.org/presenter.jhtml?identifier=3045790* ... Accessed April 6, 2010.

56. "Saturated fat," *http://www.cdc.gov/nutrition/everyone/basics/fat/saturatedfat.html* ... Accessed April 6, 2010.

57. See note 6 above, pp. 55-57.

58. "Trans fat," *http://www.cdc.gov/nutrition/everyone/basics/fat/transfat.html* ... Accessed April, 6, 2010.

59. Carper, J., "Trans fats = big bellies," *USA Weekend*, November 10-12, 2006: 4.

60. See note 6 above, pp. 55-57

61. See note 6 above, pp. 55-57.

62. "Polyunsaturated fats and monounsaturated fats," *http://www.cdc.gov/nutrition/everyone/basics/fat/unsaturatedfat.html* … Accessed April 6, 2010.

63. See note 6 above, pp. 51-54.

64. See note 6 above, pp. 55-57.

65. See note 62 above.

66. Kris-Etherton, P., Harris, W., Appel, L., "Fish consumption, fish oil, omega-3 fatty acids and cardiovascular disease," *Circulation* (2002), 31: 2747-2757.

67. McKenny, J. M., Sica, D., "Prescription omega-3 fatty acids for the treatment of hypertriglyceridemia," *Am J Health Syst Pharm* (2007); 64:595-605.

68. Park, Y., Harris, W. S., "Omega-fatty acid supplementation accelerates chylomicron triglyceride clearance," *J Lipid Res* (2004);44: 455-463.

69. Griffin, M. D., Sanders, T. A., Davies, I. G., Morgan, L. M., Millward, D. J., Lewis, F., Slaughter, S., Cooper, J. A., Miller, G. J., Griffin, B. A., "Effects of altering the ratio of n-6 to n-3 fatty acids on insulin sensitivity, lipoprotein size, and postprandial lipemia in men and post-menopausal women aged 45-70 y: The OPTILIP study," *Am J Clin Nutr* (2006);84:1290-81298.

70. See note 6 above, pp. 55-57.

71. See note 61 above.

72. "Fish 101," *http://www.americanheart.org/presenter.jhtml?identifier =3071550* … Accessed March 1, 2010.

73. "Consumer faq-"better fats (monounsaturated and polyunsatu-rated fats)," *http://www.americanheart.org/presenter.jhtml?identifier= 3046644#aha_rec_omega3* … Accessed March 1, 2010.

74. See note 6 above, pp. 55-57.

75. See note 72 above.

76. See note 6 above, pp. 55-57.

77. See note 66 above.

78. See note 67 above.

79. See note 68 above.

80. See note 69 above.

81. See note 72 above.

82. See note 73 above.

83. See note 72 above.

84. See note 66 above.

85. "What you need to know about mercury in fish and shellfish," *http://www.epa.gov/waterscience/fishadvice/advice.html* ... Accessed July 19, 2007.

86. See note 6 above, pp. 55-57.

87. See note 62 above.

88. See note 6 above, pp. 51-54.

89. See note 54 above.

90. See note 6 above, pp. 55-57.

91. Pittler, M. H., Ernst, E., "Complementary therapies for peripheral arterial disease: Systematic review," *Atherosclerosis* (2005); 181:1-7.

92. See note 6 above, pp. 51-54.

93. See note 67 above.

94. See note 73 above.

95. Mayer, K., Grimm, H., Grimminger, F., Seeger, W., "Parenteral nutrition with n-3 lipids in sepsis," *Br J Nutr* (2002);87(suppl 1):S69-S75.

96. Macdonald, A., "Omega-3 fatty acids as adjunctive therapy to Crohns disease," *Gastroenterol Nurs* (2006);29:295-301.

97. Zamaria, N., "Alteration of polyunsaturated fatty acid status and metabolism in health and disease," *Reprod Nutr Dev 44* (2004), (3):273-282.

98. "What is cholesterol?" *http://www.nhlbi.nih.gov/health/dci/Diseases/Hbc/HBC_WhatIs.html* ... Accessed April 6, 2010.

99. Thompson, G. R., Grundy, S. M., "History and development of plant sterol and stanol esters for cholesterol-lowering purposes," *Am J Cardiology* (2005); 96(1A):3D-9D.

100. Trautwein, E. A., "Proposed mechanisms of cholesterol-lowering action of plant sterols," *Eur J Lipid Sci Tech* (2003);105:171-185.

101. Bell-Wilson, J., "The power of plant sterols in cholesterol management," *Nutrition in Complementary Care* (2007);9 (4): 60.

102. Katan, M. B., Grundy, S. M., Jones, P., Law, M., Miettinen, T., Paoletti, R., "Efficacy and safety of plant stanols and sterols in the management of blood cholesterol levels," *Mayo Clin Proc* (2003);78:965-978.

103. See note 101 above.

104. See note 101 above.

105. Haynes, F., "Enova cooking oil," *http://lowfatcooking.about.com/od/healthandfitness/p/enovaoil.htm* ... Accessed November 4, 2010.

106. See note 105 above.

107. See note 6 above, pp. 51-54.

108. See note 6 above, pp. 55-57.

109. See note 6 above, pp. 51-54.

110. See note 6 above, pp. 55-57.

111. See note 98 above.

112. "What causes high blood cholesterol?" *http://www.nhlbi.nih.gov/health/dci/Diseases/Hbc/HBC_Causes.html* ... Accessed April 6, 2010.

113. "How is high blood cholesterol treated?" *http://www.nhlbi.nih.gov/health/dci/Diseases/Hbc/HBC_Treatments.html* ... Accessed April 6, 2010.

114. "High blood sugar, heart disease risk factor-diabetics and non-diabetics at increased risk," *http://www.medicalnewstoday.com/articles/30604.php* ... Accessed April 6, 2010.

115. See note 113 above.

116. "Fat," *http://www.americanheart.org/presenter.jhtml?identifier=4582* ... Accessed December 31, 2007.

117. See note 6 above, pp. 51-54.

118. See note 6 above, pp. 55-57.

Alcohol

119. See note 6 above, pp. 548.

120. See note 6 above, p. 548.

121. "Resveratrol," Oregon State University, Linus Pauling Institute Micronutrient Research for Optimum Health, *http://lpi.oregonstate.edu/infocenter/phytochemicals/resveratrol/* ... Accessed August 26, 2010.

122. Brito, P., Almeida, L. M., Dinis, T. C., "The interaction of resveratrol with ferrylmyoglobin and peroxynitrite; protection against LDL oxidation," *Free Radic Res* (2002);36(6):621-631. *(PubMed)*

123. Frankel, E. N., Waterhouse, A. L., Kinsella, J. E., "Inhibition of human LDL oxidation by resveratrol," *Lancet* (1993);341(8852):1103-1104. *(PubMed)*.

124. See note 6 above, p. 25.

125. See note 6 above, p. 548.
126. See note 6 above, p. 448.
127. Doheny, K., "FAQ: Alcohol and your health: Experts answer questions about the impact of drinking on cancer risk, heart health, and more," *http://www.webmd.com/cancer/features/faq-alcohol-and-your-health* ... Accessed April 4, 2010.
128. See note 5 above, p. 25.

Fiber

129. "Fiber fact sheet," *http://www.foodinsight.org/Content/6/FINAL %20IFICFndtnFiberFactSheet%2011%2021%2008.pdf* ... Accessed April 6, 2010.
130. "Whole grains and fiber," *http://www.americanheart.org/presenter. jhtml?identifier=4574* ... Accessed April 6, 2010.
131. Marlett, J. A., McBurney, M., Slavin, J., "Position of the American Dietetic Association: Health implications of dietary fiber," *J Am Diet Assoc* (2002);102(7):993-1000.
132. See note 129 above.
133. See note 130 above.
134. See note 131 above.
135. Aldoori, W.H., Giovannucci, E.L., Rockett, H.R., Sampson, L., Rimm, E.B., Willett, W.C., "A prospective study of dietary fiber types and symptomatic diverticular disease in men," *J Nutr* (1998);128(4): 714-9.
136. "Diverticular disease," *http://www.webmd.com/digestive-disorders/ diverticular-disease* ... Accessed December 22, 2009.
137. See note 129 above.
138. Institute of Medicine: Dietary Reference Intakes: Energy, Carbohydrate, Fiber, Fat, Fatty Acids, Cholesterol, Protein, and Amino Acids, "Dietary, Functional, and Total Fiber," pp. 339-421. Washington, DC, National Academies Press, 2002.
139. Vorvick, L. J., Zeive, D., "Position of the American Dietetic Association: Health implications of dietary fiber," *J Am Diet Assoc* (2008);108: 1716-1731.
140. See note 129 above.

Chapter 7. Exercise

Benefits

1. Hilts, P., "Exercise and longevity: A little goes a long way," *http://query.nytimes.com/gst/fullpage.html?res=950DE2D7113FF930A35742C1A 96F9482* ... April 6, 2007.

2. Chodzko-Zajko, W. J., Proctor, D. N., Fiatarone Singh, M. A., Minson, C. T., Nigg, C. R., Salem, G. J., Skinner, J. S., "Exercise and physical activity for older adults," *Medicine and Science in Sports and Exercise*, 41(7): 1510-1530, July, 2009.

3. "Measuring physical activity intensity," Centers for Disease Control and Prevention, *http://www.cdc.gov/healthyweight/physical_activity/index.html* ... Accessed March 4, 2010.

4. "Dietary guidelines for Americans 2005. Chapter 3 Weight Management," *http://www.health.gov/dietaryguidelines/dga2005/document/html/chapter3.htm#table4* ... Accessed March 5, 2010.

5. See note 2 above.

6. See note 3 above.

7. See note 4 above.

8. Duyff, R. L., *American Dietetic Association Complete Food and Nutrition Guide, 2nd Ed.* (Hoboken: John Wiley & Sons, Inc., 2002), pp. 9, 10.

9. See note 3 above.

10. See note 8 above.

10,000 Steps

11. *http://www.shapeup.org/shape/steps.php* ... Accessed February 21, 2008.

Chapter 8. Conditions Improved by Lifestyle

Arthritis

1. "Arthritis," *http://www.cdc.gov/arthritis/* ... Accessed February 20, 2010.

2. "Arthritis basics," *http://www.cdc.gov/arthritis/basics.htm* ... Accessed February 20, 2010.

3. "Most common arthritis types," *http://www.webmd.com/rheuma toid-arthritis/guide/most-common-arthritis-types* ... Accessed February 20, 2010.

4. "What is osteoarthritis?" *http://www.arthritistoday.org/conditions/ osteoarthritis/all-about-oa/what-is-oa.php* ... Accessed February 21, 2010.

5. See note 3 above.

6. See note 4 above.

7. "Osteoarthritis," *http://www.cdc.gov/arthritis/basics/osteoarthritis. htm* ... Accessed February 20, 2010.

8. Jordan, J. M., Helmick, C. G., Renner, J. B., et al., "Prevalence of knee symptoms and radiographic and symptomatic knee osteoarthritis in African Americans and Caucasians: The Johnston County Osteoarthritis Project," *J Rheumatol* (2007);34(1):172–180.

9. Felson, D. T., Zhang, Y., "An update on the epidemiology of knee and hip osteoarthritis with a view to prevention," *Arthritis Rheum* (1998); 41(8):1343–1355.

10. Felson, D. T., "Risk factors for osteoarthritis," *Clin Orthoped Rel Res* (2004);427S:S16–S21.

11. Rossignol, M., Leclerc, A., Allaert, F. A., et al., "Primary osteo- arthritis of hip, knee and hand in relation to occupational exposure," *Occup Environ Med* (2005);62:772–777.

12. "Osteoarthritis and your diet," *http://www.webmd.com/osteo arthritis/guide/osteoarthritis-diet* ... Accessed February 21, 2010.

13. OsteoarthritisfactsheetfromAF-Final2012_10_09.pdf.

14. "Rheumatoid arthritis," *http://www.cdc.gov/arthritis/basics/rheu matoid.htm* ... Accessed February 20, 2010.

15. Silman, A., "Rheumatoid arthritis," In: Silman, A., Hochberg, M. C., editors, *Epidemiology of the Rheumatic Diseases* (Oxford University Press, 2001);31–71.

16. Skarnulis, L., "Arthritis diets & supplements: Do they work?" *http://www.webmd.com/osteoarthritis/guide/arthritis-diets-supplements? page=2* ... Accessed September 23, 2005.

17. Murray M., Pizzorno J., & Pizzorno L., *The Encyclopedia of Healing Foods* (New York: Atria Books, 2005), 196.

18. Grotto, D., *101 Foods That Could Save Your Life* (New York: Bantam Dell, 2007), 250.

19. "Herbs at a glance. A quick guide to herbal supplements," U.S. Department of Health and Human Services. National Institutes of Health. National Center for Complementary and Alternative Medicine. NIH publication no. 08-6248, April 2008.

20. See note 15 above.

21. "GAIT/GUIDE study results revealed. The latest major clinical trial results are in!" *http://www.dolenutrition.com/Facts_LR.aspx* ... Accessed October 16, 2008.

22. Daniells, S., "Omega-3 plus glucosamine superior for joint health: Study," *http://www.nutraingredients-usa.com/content/view/print/268991* ... Accessed November 2009.

23. Gruenwald, J., Petzold, E., Busch, R., Petzold, H., Graubaum, J., "Effect of glucosamine sulfate with or without omega-3 fatty acids in patients with osteoarthritis," *Advances in Therapy*, 26 (9); 858-871.

24. See note 16 above, p. 99.

25. See note 16 above, p. 88.

26."Introduction to exercise," Arthritis Foundation, *http://www.arthritis.org/exercise-intro.php* ... Accessed August 26, 2010.

27. See note 16 above.

28. See note 22 above.

29. See note 23 above.

Asthma

30. "What is asthma?" *http://www.nhlbi.nih.gov/health/dci/Diseases/Asthma/Asthma_WhatIs.html* ... Accessed January 1, 2010.

31. "Asthma causes and triggers," *http://www.webmd.com/asthma/guide/asthma-triggers* ... Accessed January 1, 2010.

32. "Is obesity a risk for asthma?" *http://www.medicalnewstoday.com/articles/24118.php* ... Accessed January 1, 2010.

33. Warner, J., "Link found between asthma and GERD," *http://www.webmd.com/asthma/news/20080725/link-found-between-asthma-and-gerd* ... Accessed January 1, 2010.

34. See note 31 above.

35. "Important asthma triggers," *http://www.cdc.gov/asthma/triggers.html* ... Accessed January 1, 2010.

36. "Food allergies and asthma," *http://www.webmd.com/asthma/ guide/food-allergies-asthma* ... Accessed January 1, 2010.

37. Duyff, R. L., *American Dietetic Association Complete Food and Nutrition Guide, 2ⁿᵈ Ed.* (Hoboken: John Wiley & Sons, Inc., 2002), 524.

38. "Take control of your asthma," *http://www.lungusa.org/lung-disease/ asthma/living-with-asthma/take-control-of-your-asthma/* ... Accessed January 1, 2010.

39. Daniells, S., "Fruit and vegetable may cut adult asthma risk," *http://www.nutraingredients.com/content/view/print/18079* ... Accessed March 6, 2010.

40. Romieu, I., Trenga, C., "Diet and obstructive lung diseases," *Epidemiol Rev* (2001);23:268–287

41. Smit, H. A., Grievink, L., Tabak, C., "Dietary influences on chronic obstructive lung disease and asthma: a review of the epidemiological evidence," *Proc Nutr Soc* (1999);58:309–319

42. Painter, F. M., Coles, S. L., "Quercetin: A review of clinical applications," *http://www.chiro.org/nutrition/ABSTRACTS/Quercetin_A_ Review.shtml* ... Accessed January 1, 2010.

43. *http://www/phytochemicals.info/phytochemicals/quercetin.php* ...

44. Wong, K., "Clinical efficacy of n-3 fatty acid supplementation in patients with asthma," *J Am Diet Assoc* (2005);105:98-105.

45. Chatzi, L., Apostolaki, G., Bibakis, I., Skypala, I., Bibaki-Liakou, V., Tzanakis, N., Kogevinas, M., Cullinan, P., "Protective effect of fruits, vegetables and the Mediterranean diet on asthma and allergies among children in Crete," *Thorax* (2007);62: 677-683.

46. See note 42 above.

47. See note 43 above.

48. See note 40 above.

49. See note 41 above.

50. See note 44 above.

51. See note 45 above.

52. De Batlle, J., Garcia-Aymerich, J. G., Barraza-Villarreal, A., Anto, J. M., Romieu, I., "Mediterranean diet is associated with reduced asthma and rhinitis in Mexican children," *Allergy* (2008);63(10):1310-1316.

Cancer

53. "Understanding cancer," *http://www.cancer.gov/cancertopics/wyntk/cancer/page3* ... Accessed October 4, 2006.

54. "Defining cancer," *http://www.cancer.gov/cancertopics/what-is-cancer* ... Accessed February 20, 2008.

55. "What you need to know about cancer – risk factors," *http://www.cancer.gov/cancertopics/wyntk/overview/page4* ... Accessed October 4, 2006.

56. "The second expert report," American Institute for Cancer Research, *Science Now*, Winter, 2008: 23.

57. *http://www.cancer.org/docroot/PED/content/PED_1_3X_Infectious_Agents_and_Cancer.asp?sitearea=PED* ... Accessed October 17, 2006.

58. See note 56 above.

59. Danaei, G., Vender Horn S., Lopez A., Murray C., Ezzati M. "Causes of cancer in the world: Comparative risk assessment of nine behavior environmental risk factors," *The Lancet* (2005), 366: 1784-1793.

60. "What you need to know about cancer: Screening," *http://www.cancer.gov/cancertopics/wyntk/overview/page5* ... Accessed October 4, 2006.

61. "Newer technologies for breast cancer screening," *http://www.cancer.org/Cancer/BreastCancer/MoreInformation/BreastCancerEarlyDetection/breast-cancer-early-detection-new-screening-technologies* ... Accessed October 3, 2010.

Cardiovascular Disease

62. "What is cardiovascular disease?" *http://www.americanheart.org/presenter.jhtml?identifier=3040000* ... Accessed February 25, 2010.

63. "Cardiovascular diseases," *http://www.ynhh-healthlibrary.org/content.asp?page=P00225* ... Accessed February 25, 2010.

64. See note 63 above.

65. "What is coronary artery disease?" *http://www.nhlbi.nih.gov/health/dci/Diseases/Cad/CAD_WhatIs.html* Accessed February 25, 2010.

66. See note 63 above.

67. "Risk factors and coronary artery disease," *http://www.americanheart.org/presenter.jhtml?identifier=235* ... Accessed February 25, 2010.

68. "Who is at risk for coronary artery disease?" *http://www.nhlbi.nih.gov/health/dci/Diseases/Cad/CAD_WhoIsAtRisk.html* ... Accessed February 25, 2010.

69. See note 67 above.
70. See note 68 above.
71. See note 68 above.
72. "How is high blood cholesterol diagnosed?" *http://www.nhlbi.nih.gov/health/dci/Diseases/Hbc/HBC_Diagnosis.html* … Accessed January 1, 2008.
73. "What is cholesterol?" *http://www.nhlbi.nih.gov/health/dci/Diseases/Hbc/HBC_WhatIs.html* … Accessed January 1, 2008.
74. See note 67 above.
75. See note 68 above.
76. See note 67 above.
77. See note 68 above.
78. See note 72 above.
79. See note 67 above.
80. See note 68 above.
81. See note 68 above.
82. See note 68 above.
83. "C-reactive protein," *http://www.nlm.nih.gov/medlineplus/ency/article/003356.htm* … Accessed January 22, 2008.
84. "Inflammation, heart disease and stroke: The role of C-reactive protein," *http://www.americanheart.org/presenter.jhtml?identifier=4648* … Accessed December 2, 2009.
85. "What is homocysteine?" *http://www.americanheart.org/presenter.jhtml?identifier=535* … Accessed November 30, 2009.
86. "Heart disease and homocysteine," *http://www.webmd.com/heart-disease/guide/homocysteine-risk* … Accessed November 30, 2009.
87. "Dietary reference intakes," *http://iom.edu/en/Global/News%20Announcements/~/media/Files/Activity%20Files/Nutrition/DRIs/DRI SummaryListing2.ashx* … Accessed November 30, 2009.
88. See note 68 above.

Celiac Disease

89. Interview with Shelley Case, RD, March 4, 2010.
90. See note 89 above.
91. See note 89 above.

92. "What is celiac disease? *"http://www.digestive.niddk.nih.gov/ddiseases/pubs/celiac/#1* ... Accessed August 15, 2007.

93. Sayre, C., "The overlooked diagnosis of celiac disease," *http:// health.nytimes.com/health/healthguide/esn-celiac-ess.html?print=1* ... Accessed December 20, 2009.

94. "Digestive diseases: Celiac disease," *http://www.webmd.com/ a-to-z-guides/celiac-disease* ... Accessed March 1, 2006.

95. See note 89 above.

96. See note 92 above.

97. See note 93 above.

98. See note 89 above.

99. See note 92 above.

100. See note 93 above.

101. See note 94 above.

102. See note 89 above.

103. See note 89 above.

104. See note 92 above.

105. See note 93 above.

106. See note 94 above.

107. See note 93 above.

108. See note 89 above.

109. See note 92 above.

110. See note 89 above.

111. See note 89 above.

112. See note 93 above.

113. See note 89 above.

114. See note 92 above.

Dental Hygiene

115. Nazario, B., "Healthy mouth, healthy body? The impact of teeth, breath, and gum problems. The mouth-body connection: 6 ways oral hygiene helps keep you well," *http://www.webmd.com/oral-health/healthy-mouth-and-body-9/gum-disease-health?page=1* ... Accessed August 5, 2010.

116. "Oral health preventing cavities, gum disease, tooth loss, and oral cancers: At a glance 2010," *http://www.cdc.gov/chronicdisease/resources/publications/AAG/doh.htm* ... Accessed August 4, 2010.

117. "Diet and oral health," *http://www.webmd.com/oral-health/guide/ diet-oral-health* ... Accessed August 26, 2010.

118. Daniells, S., "Green tea may boost oral health, reduce tooth loss," *http://www.nutraingredients.com/Research/Green-tea-may-boost-oral- health-reduce-tooth-loss* ... Accessed August 26, 2010.

119. See note 117 above.

120. Daniells, S., "Omega-3 may combat mouth bacteria, boost oral health," *http://www.nutraingredients.com/Research/Omega-3-may-combat- mouth-bacteria-boost-oral-health* ... Accessed August 26, 2010.

121. Huang, C. B., Ebersole, J. L., "A novel bioactivity of omega-3 polyunsaturated fatty acids and their ester derivatives," *Molecular Oral Microbiology* (2010);25(1): 75-80.

Diabetes

122. "The facts about diabetes: America's seventh leading cause of death," *http://www.ndep.nih.gov/diabetes-facts/index.aspx#whatisdiabetes* ... Accessed April 3, 2010.

123. See note 31 above, p. 559.

124. "Diagnosis of diabetes," *http://diabetes.niddk.nih.gov/dm/pubs/ diagnosis/* ... Accessed April 3, 2010.

125. See note 31 above, p. 559.

126. See note 124 above.

127. "Protect your heart against diabetes," *http://www.nhlbi.nih.gov/ health/public/heart/other/latino/diabetes/* ... Accessed April 3, 2010.

128. "Manage diabetes," *http://www.nhlbi.nih.gov/actintime/rhar/md. htm* ... Accessed April 3, 2010.

129. See note 122 above.

130. See note 31 above, p. 559.

131. See note 124 above.

132. See note 127 above.

133. See note 128 above.

134. See note 124 above.

135. See note 124 above.

136. See note 124 above.

137. "Diabetes overview," *http://diabetes.niddk.nih.gov/dm/pubs/over view/index.htm#types* ... Accessed April 3, 2010.

138. "Diabetes basics," *http://www.diabetes.org/diabetes-basics/type-1/* ... Accessed April 3, 2010.

139. See note 138 above.

140. See note 137 above.

141. See note 138 above.

142. See note 128 above.

143. See note 137 above.

144. See note 138 above.

145. See note 124 above.

146. "Diabetes basics," *http://www.diabetes.org/diabetes-basics/type-2/* ... Accessed April 3, 2010.

147. Peckenpaugh, N., *Nutrition Essentials and Diet Therapy, 10th Ed.,* (Amsterdam: Elsevier, 2007), 232.

148. See note 128 above.

149. See note 146 above.

150. Parillo, M., Riccardi, G., "Diet composition and the risk of type 2 diabetes: Epidemiological and clinical evidence," *Br J Nutr* (2004);92(1): 7-19.

151. See note 128 above.

152. See note 150 above.

153. "For warding off diabetes, magnesium," *Tufts Health and Nutrition Letter* (2004);22(4):1.

154. "Chromium – topic overview," *http://www.webmd.com/balance/tc/Chromium-Topic-Overview* ... Accessed June 27, 2007.

155. DRI report—vitamin A vitamin K, arsenic, boron, chromium, copper, iodine, iron, manganese, molybdenum, nickel, silicon, vanadium, and zinc, *http://fnic.nal.usda.gov/nal_display/index.php?info_center=4&tax_level=4&tax_subject=256&topic_id=1342&level3_id=5141&level4_id =10590* ... Accessed March 6, 2010.

156. Anderson, R. A., Cheng, N., Bryden, N. A., et al. "Elevated intakes of supplemental chromium improve glucose and insulin variables in individuals with type 2 diabetes," *Diabetes* (1997);46:1786-91.

157. Althius, M. D., Jordon, N. E., Ludington, E. A., Wittes, J. T., "Glucose and insulin responses to dietary chromium supplements: A meta-analysis," *Am J Clin Nutr* (2003);76:148-55.

158. Anderson, R. A., "Chromium, glucose intolerance and diabetes," *J Am Col Nutrition* (1998);17(6): 548-555.

159. See note 155 above.

160. See note 155 above.

161. See note 156 above.

162. See note 157 above.

163. See note 158 above.

164. Willet, W., *Self,* February (2006):90.

165. See note 78 above, p. 243.

166. See note 31 above, p. 443.

167. Heller, L., "FDA awaits stevia petition," *Food Navigator USA, http://www.foodnavigator-usa.com/news/printNewsBis.asp?id=80248 ...* Accessed October 2, 2007.

168. See note 31 above, p. 125.

169. Hitti, M., "Cinnamon may prove useful for diabetes, spice's ingredients might help control blood sugar; no food prescription yet," *http://diabetes.webmd.com/news/20060404/cinnamon-may-prove-useful-for-diabetes ...* Accessed April 4, 2006.

170. See note 16 above, pp. 98-101.

171. Neville, K., "Spice up your health: some seasonings carry antioxidant benefits as well as wonderful flavor," *http://www.chicagotribune. com/features/food/chi-0609130054sep13,1,179195.story?coll ...* Accessed September 14, 2006.

172. See note 171 above.

173. See note 169 above.

174. Johnston, C., Buller, A., "Vinegar and peanut products as complementary foods to reduce postprandial glycemia," *J Am Diet Assoc* (2005);105(12):1939-1942.

Eye Health

175. "Eye Disease," *http://www.geteyesmart.org/eyesmart/diseases/ index.cfm ...* Accessed April 11, 2010.

176. See note 175 above.

177. Reader's Digest Association, Inc., *The Healing Power of Vitamins, Minerals, and Herbs,* (Pleasantville: Friedman, 1999), 80.

178. "Cataract: What you should know," *http://www.nei.nih.gov/health/cataract/webcataract.pdf* ... Accessed April 11, 2010.

179. See note 175 above.

180. See note 177 above.

181. See note 178 above.

182. See note 175 above.

183. See note 177 above.

184. See note 178 above.

185. Bauer, J., *Food Cures*, (New York: Rodale, 2007), 255-264.

186. DeNoon, D. J., "Cataracts from antidepressants? Study: 22,000 U.S. cataract cases may be due to SSRI antidepressants," *http://www.webmd.com/eye-health/cataracts/news/20100312/cataracts-from-antidepressants* ... Accessed April 11, 2010.

187. See note 186 above.

188. See note 175 above.

189. See note 178 above.

190. See note 175 above.

191. See note 177 above.

192. See note 178 above.

193. See note 185 above.

194. See note 186 above.

195. Carper, J., "Super foods for eyes," *USA Weekend*, June 16-18, (2006):12.

196. See note 175 above.

197. "Facts about dry eye," *http://www.nei.nih.gov/health/dryeye/dryeye.asp#5* ... Accessed April 11, 2010.

198. "Dry eye," *http://www.geteyesmart.org/eyesmart/diseases/dry-eye-cause.cfm* ... Accessed April 11, 2010.

199. "Dry eyes," *http://www.webmd.com/eye-health/eye-health-dry-eyes* ... Accessed April 11, 2010.

200. See note 195 above.

201. See note 196 above.

202. See note 185 above.

203. See note 199 above.

204. See note 199 above.

205. "Age-related macular degeneration., *http://www.geteyesmart.org/ eyesmart/diseases/amd.cfm* ... Accessed April 11, 2010.

206. See note 199 above.

207. See note 177 above.

208. See note 205 above.

209. See note 177 above.

210. See note 199 above.

211. See note 205 above.

212. See note 185 above.

213. See note 199 above.

214. See note 205 above.

215. "Facts about age-related macular degeneration," *http://www.nei. nih.gov/health/maculardegen/armd_facts.asp* ... Accessed April 11, 2010.

216. See note 205 above.

217. See note 185 above.

218. See note 185 above.

219. See note 195 above.

220. "Age-related eye disease study-results," *http://www.nei.nih.gov/ amd/* ... Accessed April 11, 2010.

221. "DHA: A good fat," Nutrition Fact Sheet, American Dietetic Association, 2008.

GERD

222. "GERD," *http://www.mayoclinic.com/health/gerd/DS00967* ... Accessed April 10, 2010.

223. "Heartburn, gastroesophageal reflux (GER), and gastroesophageal reflux disease (GERD)," *http://digestive.niddk.nih.gov/ddiseases/pubs/gerd/* ... Accessed April 10, 2010.

224. "Gastroesophageal reflux (GERD) & laryngopharyngeal reflux (LPR)," *http://www.entnet.org/HealthInformation/GERD-and-LPR.cfm* ... Accessed April 10, 2010.

225. See note 222 above.

226. See note 223 above.

227. See note 224 above.

228. See note 222 above.

229. See note 223 above.

230. Jacobson, B., Somers, S., Fuchs, C., Kelly, C., Camargo, C., "Body-mass index and symptoms of gastroesophageal reflux in women," *New England Journal of Medicine* (2006);354:2340-2348.

231. See note 222 above.

232. See note 223 above.

233. See note 224 above.

234. DeNoon, D., "Acid-reflux drugs may up fractures, proton pump inhibitors—the popular drugs that fight stomach acid—increase the risk of hip fractures, a U.S. study shows," WebMD Medical News, *http://www.webmd.com/heartburn-gerd/news/20061227/acid-reflux-drugs-may-up-fractures* ... December 26, 2006.

235. Hyman, M., *The Ultramind Solution* (New York: Scribner, 2009), 212-214.

236. Ruscin, J. M., Page, R. L., Valuck, R. J., "Vitamin B_{12} deficiency associated with histamine(2)-receptor antagonists and a proton-pump inhibitor," *Ann Pharmacother* (2002);36 (5):812-816.

High Blood Pressure/Hypertension

237. "What is high blood pressure?" *http://www.nhlbi.nih.gov/health/dci/Diseases/Hbp/HBP_WhatIs.html* ... Accessed January 1, 2008.

238. See note 237 above.

239. Kotchen, T., McCarron, D. A., "Dietary electrolytes and blood pressure: A statement for healthcare professionals from the American Heart Association nutrition committee," *Circulation* (1998);98:613-617.

240. See note 31 above, pp. 144-152.

241. "Sodium (salt or sodium chloride)," *http://www.americanheart.org/presenter.jhtml?identifier=4708* ... Accessed April 8, 2010.

242. "Add potassium to help lower blood pressure. Nutrition Fact Sheet," American Dietetic Association, 2008.

243. See note 241 above.

Metabolic Syndrome

244. "What is metabolic syndrome?" *http://www.nhlbi.nih.gov/health/dci/Diseases/ms/ms_whatis.html* ... Accessed April 9, 2010.

245. See note 78 above, pp. 152-153.

246. See note 244 above.

247. "Metabolic syndrome," *http://www.americanheart.org/presenter.jhtml?identifier=4756* ... Accessed April 9, 2010.

248. "Metabolic syndrome," *http://www.mayoclinic.com/health/metabolic%20syndrome/DS00522/DSECTION=risk-factors* ... Accessed April 9, 2010.

249. "Metabolic syndrome-topic overview," *http://www.webmd.com/heart/metabolic-syndrome/tc/metabolic-syndrome-topic-overview* ... Accessed April 9, 2010.

250. Cowey, S., Hardy, R. W., "The metabolic syndrome: A high risk state for cancer?" *American Journal of Pathology* (2006);169:1505-1522.

251. Stocks, T., Borena, W., Strohmaier, S., Bjorge, T., Manjer, J., Engeland, A., Johansen, D., Selmer, R., Hallmans, G., Rapp, K., et al., "Cohort profile: The metabolic syndrome and cancer project (Me-Can)," *Int. J. Epidemiol,* April 20, 2009; dyp186v1.

252. See note 244 above.

253. See note 247 above.

254. See note 248 above.

255. See note 249 above.

256. See note 250 above.

257. See note 251 above.

258. Rose, D. P., Haffner, S. M., Baillargeon, J., "Adiposity, the metabolic syndrome, and breast cancer in African-American and white American women," *Endocrine Reviews* (2007);28(7):763-777.

259. See note 244 above.

260. See note 248 above.

Osteoporosis

261. "Osteoporosis facts," Best bones forever! Act now. US Department of Health and Human Services, *http://www.bestbonesforever.gov/parents/osteoporosis/tips.cfm* ... Accessed June 1, 2010.

262. "Understanding osteoporosis," *http://women.webmd.com/guide/understanding-osteoporosis-basics* ... Accessed June 1, 2009.

263. "What is osteoporosis?" *http://womensguide.org/osteoporosis/overview.html?utm_medium=ppc&utm_source=b2345y1007&utm_campaign=wg_osteo_general&utm_content=osteopenia&OVRAW=Osteopenia&OV*

KEY=osteopenia&OVMTC=standard&OVADID=1443341012&OVKWID=11271429512 ... Accessed June 2, 2009.

264. "Osteoporosis," *http://www.niams.nih.gov/Health_Info/Bone/Osteoporosis/default.asp#a* ... Accessed June 2, 2009.

265. See note 261 above.

266. See note 262 above.

267. See note 263 above.

268. See note 264 above.

269. See note 264 above.

270. See note 261 above.

271. See note 262 above.

272. See note 263 above.

273. See note 264 above.

274. See note 261 above

275. See note 262 above.

276. See note 263 above.

277. See note 264 above.

278. "Osteopenia-overview," *http://www.webmd.com/osteoporosis/tc/osteopenia-overview* ... Accessed April 10, 2010.

279. See note 261 above.

280. See note 262 above.

281. See note 263 above.

282. See note 264 above.

283. See note 278 above.

284. "Osteoporosis prevention," *http://www.nof.org/prevention/index.htm* ... Accessed April 10, 2010.

285. Gallagher, J. C., Goldgar, D., Moy, A., "Total bone calcium in normal women: effect of age and menopause status," *J Bone Min Res* (1987); 2:491-6. [*PubMed abstract*]

286. Heaney, R. P., Recker, R. R., Stegman, M. R., Moy, A. J., "Calcium absorption in women: Relationships to calcium intake, estrogen status, and age," *J Bone Miner Res* (1989);4:469-75. [*PubMed abstract*]

287. Breslau, N. A., "Calcium, estrogen, and progestin in the treatment of osteoporosis," *Rheum Dis Clin North Am* (1994);20:691-716. [*PubMed abstract*]

288. Gallagher, J. C., Riggs, B. L., Deluca, H. F., "Effect of estrogen on

calcium absorption and serum vitamin D metabolites in postmenopausal osteoporosis," *J Clin Endocrinol Metab* (1980); 51:1359-64. [*PubMed abstract*]

289. Gregg, E. W., et al., "Physical activity, falls, and fractures among older adults: A review of the epidemiologic evidence," *Am. Geriatric Soc* (2000); 48:888-893.

290. "What you should know about calcium," National Osteoporosis Foundation, *http://www.nof.org/prevention/calcium2.htm* ... Accessed March 5, 2010.

291. Dietary Supplement Fact Sheet: Calcium. National Institutes of Health Office of Dietary Supplements, *http://dietary-supplements.info.nih.gov/factsheets/calcium.asp* ... Accessed March 6, 2010.

292. "Vitamin D for Osteoporosis," *http://www.webmd.com/osteoporosis/guide/vitamin-d-for-osteoporosis* ... July 7, 2005.

293. Weiss, L., Barrett-Connor, E., von Muhlen, D., "Ratio of n-6 to n-3 fatty acids and bone mineral density in older adults: The Rancho Bernardo Study," *Am J Clin Nutr* (2005); 81 (4):934-938.

294. Vitamin K, *http://www.vitamins-supplements.org/vitamin-K.php* ... Accessed July 20, 2008.

295. Pizzorno, L., "Vitamin K-keeping calcium in your bones and out of your blood vessels," *http://blogs.webmd.com/integrative-medicine-wellness/2007/11/vitamin-k-keeping-calcium-in-your-bones.html* ... Accessed July 20, 2008.

296. "Other nutrients and bone health at a glance." *http://www.niams.nih.gov/Health_Info/Bone/Bone_Health/Nutrition/other_nutrients.asp* ... Accessed July 20, 2008.

297. "Magnesium," Reviewed by J. Goldstone, *http://www.webmd.com/diet/vitamins-supplements-8/supplement-guide-magnesium* ... Accessed July 20, 2008.

298. "Food labeling: Health claims; calcium and osteoporosis, and calcium, vitamin D, and osteoporosis," U.S. Food and Drug Administration, *http://www.fda.gov/Food/LabelingNutrition/LabelClaims/HealthClaimsMeetingSignificantScientificAgreementSSA/default.htm* ... Accessed April 20, 2010.

299. Bhattacharyaa, A., Rahmana, M., Suna, D., Fernandes, G., "Effect of fish oil on bone mineral density in aging C57BL/6 female mice," *J Nutr Biochem* (2007); 18(6):372-379.

300. See note 299 above.

301. Weaver, C. M., Heaney, R. P., "Calcium." In: Shils, M. E., Shike, M., Ross, A. C., Caballero, B., Cousins, R. J., *Modern Nutrition in Health and Disease, 10th ed*" (Baltimore: Lippincott Williams & Wilkins, 2006),194-210.

302. See note 291 above.

303. See note 290 above.

304. See note 289 above.

305. See note 297 above.

306. See note 294 above.

307. See note 295 above.

308. See note 296 above.

309. See note 296 above.

310. See note 296 above.

311. See note 297 above.

312. See note 296 above.

313. See note 296 above.

Hormonal Changes, Appetite and Mood

314. Brizendine, L., "Beating hormonal weight gain," *More*, July/August (2007): 210-216.

315. Bouchez, C., "Escape from hormone horrors—what you can do," *http://women.webmd.com/features/escape-hormone-horrors-what-you-can-do* ... Accessed April 3, 2010.

316. "Male menopause," *http://men.webmd.com/guide/male-menopause* ... Accessed April 3, 2010.

317. Monti, V., Carlson, J. J., Hunt, S. C., Adams, T. D., "Relationship of ghrelin and leptin hormones with body mass index and waist circumference in a random sample of adults," *J Am Diet Assoc* (2006);106(6):822-828.

318. Caro, J. F., Kolaczynski, J. W., Nyce, M. R., Ohannesian, J. P., Opentanova, I., Goldman, W. H., Lynn, R. B., Zhang, P. L., Sinha, M. K., Considine, R. V., "Decreased cerebrospinal fluid/serum leptin ration in obesity: A possible mechanism for leptin resistance," *Lancet* (1996); 348:159-161.

319. "Definition of dopamine," *http://www.medterms.com/script/main/art.asp?articlekey=14345* ... Accessed April 10, 2010.

320. "Dopamine-A sample neurotransmitter," *http://www.utexas.edu/research/asrec/dopamine.html* ... Accessed April 10, 2010.

321. See note 314 above

322. See note 317 above.

323. See note 318 above.

324. Altman, J., "Weight in the balance," *Neuroendocrinology* (2002); 76:131-136.

325. See note 314 above.

326. "Sleep: Fact or fiction?" *http://www.webmd.com/sleep-disorders/guide/sleep-fact-fiction* ... Accessed April 10, 2010.

327. See note 314 above.

328. "Cortisol review: What you should know," *http://www.vitalhealthpartners.com/cortisol-review/* ... Accessed April 10, 2010.

329. See note 315 above.

330. See note 316 above.

331. Hoffman, M., "Low testosterone: How to talk to your doctor," *http://men.webmd.com/features/low-testosterone-how-to-talk-to-your-doctor* Accessed April 10, 2010.

332. See note 314 above.

Sleep Disorders

333. "Your guide to healthy sleep," *http://www,nhlbi.nih.gov/health/public/sleep/healthy_sleep.pdf* ... Accessed August 27, 2010

334. "What is sleep?" American Sleep Association, *http://www.sleepassociation.org/index.php?p=whatissleep* ... Accessed August 27, 2010.

335. See note 333 above.

336. "Sleep: Fact or fiction?" *http://www.webmd.com/sleep-disorders/guide/sleep-fact-fiction* ... Accessed August 27, 2010.

337. See note 333 above.

338. See note 334 above.

339. See note 336 above.

340. See note 333 above.

341. See note 333 above.

342. See note 334 above.

343. See note 334 above.

344. See note 333 above.

345. "Insomnia," *http://www.mayoclinic.com/health/insomnia/DS00187/ DSECTION=complications* ... Accessed April 10, 2010.

346. See note 333 above.

347. See note 345 above.

348. Lewith, G. T., Godfrey, A. D., Prescott, P., "A single blinded, randomized pilot study evaluating the aroma of Lavandula augustofolia as a treatment for mild insomnia," *J of Alternative and Complementary Medicine* (2005);11(4) 631-637.

Sleep Apnea

349. "Your guide to healthy sleep," *http://www.nhlbi.nih.gov/health/ public/sleep/healthy_sleep.pdf* , p. 40-49.

350. "What is sleep?" American Sleep Association, *http://www.sleep association.org/index.php?p=whatissleep* ... Accessed August 27, 2010.

351. "Sleep: Fact or fiction?" *http://www.webmd.com/sleep-disorders/ guide/sleep-fact-fiction* ... Accessed August 27, 2010.

352. See note 349 above.

353. See note 350 above.

354. See note 351 above.

355. See note 349 above,

356. See note 350 above.

357. See note 351 above.

358. See note 349 above,

359. See note 350 above.

360. See note 349 above.

361. See note 350 above.

362. See note 351 above.

Got the Blues and No Rhythm?

363. Stambor, Z., "Stressed out nation: Many Americans resort to unhealthy habits to manage extreme stress a new survey suggests," *http:// www.apa.org/monitor/apr06/nation.aspx* ... Accessed April 4, 2010.

364. Sisk, J., "Exercise to stamp out stress," *Today's Dietitian*, June, (2006):82.

365. Hilts, P., "Exercise and longevity: A little goes a long way," *http:/ /query.nytimes.com/gst/fullpage.html?res=950DE2D7113FF930A35742C1A 96F9482* ... April 6, 2007.

366. Chodzko-Zajko, W. J., Proctor, D. N., Fiatarone Singh, M. A., Minson, C. T., Nigg, C. R., Salem, G. J., Skinner, J. S., "Exercise and physical activity for older adults," *Medicine and Science in Sports and Exercise* (2009);41(7):1510-1530.

367. Hoogendijk, W. J .G., Lips, P., Dik, M. G., Deeg, D. J. H., Beekman, A. T. F., Penninx, B. W. J. H., "Depression is associated with decreased 25-Hydroxyvitamin D and increased parathyroid hormone levels in older adults," *Archives of General Psychiatry* (2008);65(5):508-512.

368. "Omega-3 fatty acids influence mood, impulsivity, and personality, study indicates," *http://www.sciencedaily.com/releases/2006/03/06030320 5050.htm* ... Accessed March 27, 2010.

369. Harding, A., "Fatty acid tied to depression and inflammation," *http://www.reuters.com/article/idUSCOL76158120070417* ... Accessed August 27, 2010.

Skin Care

370. "Skin problems & treatments health center," *http://www.webmd. com/skin-problems-and-treatments/picture-of-the-skin* ... Accessed May 31, 2010.

371. "Dermatologists' top tips for healthy skin, hair and nails," *http:// www.aad.org/public/conditions/_doc/TopTipsforSkinHairandNails.htm* ... Accessed May 31, 2010.

372. Bender, M., "Want skin like a doctor?" *http://www.more.com/ 2018/10902-secrets-of-dermatologists* ... Accessed June 15, 2010.

373. Helfrich, Y. R., Sachs, D. L., Voorhees, J. J., "Overview of skin aging and photoaging," *Dermatology Nursing*, 2008;20(3):177-183.

374. Landau, M. D., "Is sugar aging you?" *http://www.more.com/2030/ 6242-is-sugar-bad-for-you* ... Accessed May 31, 2010.

375. Baumann, L., "Too much sugar causes wrinkles," *http://health. yahoo.com/experts/skintype/15198/too-much-sugar-causes-wrinkles/print/* ... Accessed March 21, 2010.

376. Janes, B., "The great skin diet," *http://www.self.com/beauty/2008/ 10/clear-skin-diet* ... Accessed May 31, 2010.

377. "Ask the expert: Does smoking make skin cancer worse?" *http:// www.skincancer.org/ask-the-expert-does-smoking-make-skin-cancer-worse. html* ... Accessed May 31, 2010.

378. See note 371 above.

379. See note 372 above.

380. See note 373 above.

381. See note 375 above.

382. See note 374 above.

383. See note 376 above.

384. See note 372 above.

385. See note 376 above.

386. "Vitamin C," *http://www.nlm.nih.gov/medlineplus/ency/article/002404.htm* ... Accessed May 31, 2010.

387. "Get rich on vitamin E," *http://www.eatright.org/Public/content.aspx?id=3834&terms=skin+health* ... Accessed May 31, 2010.

388. "Vitamin A," *http://www.nlm.nih.gov/medlineplus/ency/article/002400.htm* ... Accessed May 31, 2010.

389. Heinrich, U., Neukam, K., Tronnier, H., Sies, H, Stahl, W., "Long-term ingestion of high flavanol cocoa provides photoprotection against UV-induced erythema and improves skin condition in women," *Nutr* (2006);136:1565-1569.

390. Bouchez, C., "23 ways to reduce wrinkles: Worried that your skin looks older than you feel? Here are 23 ways to reduce wrinkles—starting now!" *http://www.webmd.com/skin-beauty/features/23-ways-to-reduce-wrinkles* ... Accessed June 2, 2010.

391. "Iron in Diet," *http://www.nlm.nih.gov/medlineplus/ency/article/002422.htm* ... Accessed June 2, 2010.

392. See note 390 above.

Index

fat, *continued*
  saturated, 61, 72, 109, 112-13,
    119-21, 126, 139, 155, 157
fatty acids, 112, 114, 118, 144, 170
Fenster, Carol, 166-7
fiber, 6, 15, 64, 66, 73, 75, 87, 89,
    93-4, 96, 102, 104-7, 110,
    119, 123-6, 179
  insoluble, 70, 124, 149
  soluble, 70, 124, 157
fiber intake, 15, 123, 125
fish, 46, 54, 77, 110, 115-16, 142,
    144, 193, 196, 200-1
  canned, 67, 71
flashes, hot, 13, 208
flax, 115, 144
flour, 54, 61-2, 96, 129, 165, 205
fluid retention, 101, 191, 193
fluids, 14-15, 59, 183, 191, 217
folic acid, 160
food allergies, 25, 27, 29, 31, 33,
    35, 37, 39, 41, 43, 45, 47, 49,
    51-3, 55, 57
Food and Drug Administration
    (FDA), 26-30, 35, 54, 116,
    200-1
food intolerances, 53, 55, 84
food labels, 28, 35, 53-4
food sensitivities, 55-7
foodborne illness, 75-7
foods, 5-9, 15-18, 34-5, 42-6, 49-
    52, 56, 59-61, 73-9, 85-8,
    90-6, 104-6, 123, 140-1, 143-
    4, 148-9, 172-5
  cold, 77
  fortified, 34, 40, 160, 200, 203

fried, 48, 113, 120
  healthier, 7
  healthy, 59, 86
  healthy soluble fiber, 177
  high fiber, 173
  low sodium, 192
  organic, 6
  processed, 105, 193, 202, 214
  spoilage of, 9
  sugary, 210, 216
fortified food, 6, 75
fractures, 198-9
fructose, 73, 105-6, 157
fruit, 7, 15, 44, 48, 61, 63, 65, 67,
    73, 96, 105, 107, 123-4, 126,
    144, 179
  juices, 64, 73, 106-7
functional foods, 8, 10, 50

G

garlic, 40, 66, 69, 153, 178, 185-6,
    205
GERD (Gastroesophageal Reflux
    Disease), 143, 187-8, 209
ghrelin, 206-7
ginger, 45, 47-8, 141, 152-3, 177,
    186-7
glucose, 59, 73, 104-8, 159, 170-2,
    174
gluten, 60, 162-5
glycerol, 112, 118
grains, 15, 40, 50, 63, 68, 71, 73,
    104, 107, 110, 126, 139, 144,
    162, 177, 196
green leafy vegetables, 160, 181,
    191, 200, 202-3, 217

supplements, 6, 13-15, 21, 23, 25-7, 29-35, 37, 39, 41, 43-5, 47, 49, 51, 53, 142, 164-5

sweets, 70, 92, 96, 106, 176, 186, 191

T

tacos, 67-9

tea, green, 31-2, 44, 93, 154, 169, 181, 216

teeth, 93, 167-9, 174, 200

television, 1, 12, 87, 135, 210

telomere, 31

textured vegetable protein (TVP), 64, 103

tobacco, 42, 141, 147, 168-9

tooth decay, 168-9

total cholesterol (TC), 156

toxicity, 37-8

trainers, 23

trans fats, 113-14, 118, 121

triglycerides, 84, 114, 118, 156-7, 175

tryptophan, 109-10

5-Hydroxytryptophan (5-HTP), 55

turmeric, 44-5, 47-8, 66, 68, 70, 96, 141-2, 177, 205

U

U.S. Pharmacopeia (USP), 30

UV energy, 34

UV radiation, 36

UV sunlight exposure, 180

UVA and UVB radiation, 36

UVA and UVB rays, 216

V

valerian, 211

vegetables, 7, 15, 42, 44, 48, 50, 62-5, 67, 73, 104-5, 123-4, 144, 153, 187, 191-2, 205

vegetarian products, 103

vegetarianism, 16

vinegar, 47, 64, 66-7, 110, 142, 153, 162, 166, 177, 192, 200

virus, 143, 172

vision, 180, 182-3

blurred, 171, 183

central, 182-3

healthy, 50

vision loss, 170, 182, 184

vitamin, 5, 10, 27-8, 31-8, 43-5, 51, 60, 70-1, 73, 75, 160, 181-2, 184, 200-3, 214, 216-18

essential, 25, 106, 182

fat soluble, 10, 33, 112

vitamin B6, 110

vitamin B12, 189

vitamin D2, 33-4

vitamin D3, 33-4, 36

VLDL (Very Low Density Lipoprotein), 84

vodka/gin/rum, 123

vomiting, 37, 51, 162

W

waist circumference, 100

waistline, 195

walnuts, 34, 113, 144, 146, 186,
198
water, 5, 30, 35, 63, 73, 76-7, 94,
97-8, 101, 107-8, 125-6, 146,
161, 166, 169-70, 217
fluoridated, 168
weakness, unexplained, 171
weight, 2, 73, 83-5, 90, 114, 131,
133, 136, 141, 148, 175, 181,
184, 188, 193, 199-200
excess, 159, 173
healthy, 84, 139, 188, 190
losing, 83
weight loss, 5, 83, 100, 111, 134,
171, 196
desired, 83
healthy, 132
weight-loss packages, 84
weight maintenance, 131
weight management, 95, 140
weight training techniques, 133
Weil, Andrew, 42
wellness, 1, 3, 84
Western type diet, 109
Wet AMD (age-related macular
degeneration), 183

wheat, 34-3, 107, 124-6, 163, 163
wheat intolerance, 55
wheat starch, 164
whole grains, 15, 40, 50, 63, 73,
107, 110, 126, 139, 144, 177,
202
wine, 49, 94, 122, 194, 196
worker productivity, 3
wound healing, 10, 170, 215

X

x-rays, 147, 150-1, 199
xanthan gum, 166
Xenical, 38
xylitol, 74, 176

Y

yeast, 166, 170
yoga, 133, 135, 214
yogurt, 34-5, 39-40, 42, 60, 89,
143, 179, 191, 206

Z

zeaxanthin, 45, 182, 185-7
zinc, 43, 184-7, 204, 217
zinc oxide, 216

About the Author

Susan Piergeorge is a registered dietitian (RD). At a young age, she became interested in the role food and nutrition play in health. Her father was a physician and her mother was a nurse, so medicine was a regular conversation at the dinner table. She also helped her mother in the kitchen and enjoyed cooking.

Susan saw a number of her relatives live with the challenges from conditions such as diabetes, cancer, heart disease, and arthritis. She realized that taking care of one's health could play a large role in fending off the onset and severity of these conditions.

She became an RD and worked in many clinical specialty areas including cancer (oncology), cardiovascular disease, diabetes, nutrition support, and preventive nutrition. She saw many people improve their health and quality of life from simple lifestyle changes. While working in the hospital setting she was called upon to assist with patient menu revisions. This led to her acquiring a professional culinary certificate.

Susan also worked as a health education coordinator and developed and presented a number of programs including work-site wellness, nutrition, smoking cessation, stress management, and cardiopulmonary resuscitation (CPR). She has also worked in the food manufacturing industry, learning the business, sales, and marketing aspects of the trade.

Susan has received awards from organizations such as the American Diabetes Association, American Heart Association and American Cancer Society for her volunteer efforts and community outreach.

She enjoys outdoor activities, cooking, traveling, and music.

Susan is available for speaking engagements and culinary demonstrations.
You can reach her at *susan@susanpiergeorge.com*
Her website is *www.susanpiergeorge.com*

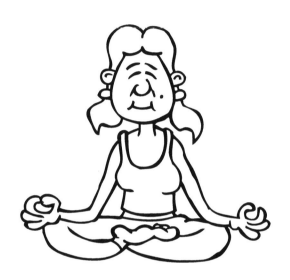